SOUPING
IS THE
NEW
JUICING

SOUPING
IS THE
NEW
JUICING

Cherie Calbom, MS

SILOAM

Most CHARISMA HOUSE BOOK GROUP products are available at special quantity discounts for bulk purchase for sales promotions, premiums, fund-raising, and educational needs. For details, write Charisma House Book Group, 600 Rinehart Road, Lake Mary, Florida 32746, or telephone (407) 333-0600.

SOUPING IS THE NEW JUICING by Cherie Calbom, MS
Published by Siloam
Charisma Media/Charisma House Book Group
600 Rinehart Road
Lake Mary, Florida 32746
www.charismahouse.com

Cover design by Lisa Rae McClure
Design Director: Justin Evans

Visit the author's websites at www.juiceladycherie.com and www.soupsbycherie.com.

Library of Congress Cataloging-in-Publication Data:
Names: Calbom, Cherie, author.
Title: Souping is the new juicing / by Cherie Calbom, MS.
Description: Lake Mary, Florida : Siloam, 2017. | Includes bibliographical
   references.
Identifiers: LCCN 2017029041| ISBN 9781629994659 (trade paper) | ISBN
   9781629994666 (ebook)

Subjects: SLCSH: Soups--Therapeutic use. | Detoxification
(Health) | Reducing
    diets.
Classification: LCC RM219 .C23 2017 | DDC 613.2--dc23
LC record available at https://lccn.loc.gov/2017029041

17 18 19 20 21 — 9 8 7 6 5 4 3 2 1
Printed in the United States of America

CONTENTS

ACKNOWLEDGMENTS

I WANT TO EXPRESS my deep and lasting appreciation to Robin Phillips and Kathryn Proa, who helped me with writing and research for this book. I also want to thank Chef Jeff McGee for developing a number of unique recipes for this book.

A sincere thank-you goes to my editor, Megan Turner.

Much thanks to my agent, Pamela Harty, for her help, guidance, and listening ear. How blessed I have been.

Finally, my deep gratitude and continued appreciation to Fr. John, my husband and official soup taster. And to my heavenly Father, who has always guided my life and healed my body and soul.

INTRODUCTION

*If someone makes you
soup, they love you.*

—UNKNOWN

SOUPING, THE NEW craze in town, often refers to making a blended drink or raw soup, and it is a way to cleanse your body and lose weight. When souping, you can make blended raw soups as mentioned above, and these soups provide fiber, biophotons, enzymes, and vitamins. Some people actually call these concoctions "juice," hence our title, *Souping Is the New Juicing*. Souping also encompasses making gently warmed soups and the old-fashioned stove-top-simmered hot soup.

Soup can be a great part of a cleanse program. Raw blended soups can give you more substance during a fast, and warm soups are especially helpful in the winter when you need something to take the chill off your body and soul or something more substantial than a glass of clear juice. You can eat just soup or soup and fresh juices throughout the day. You'll cleanse right down to your cells. I'm all for that since I've been promoting detoxification for a couple decades. But even though souping is great for cleanses and detoxes, I actually see souping as a way of life; it is not just a trend or something you do when you want to lose a few pounds or detox.

According to Dr. Nada Milosavljevic, the director of the Integrative Health Program at Massachusetts General Hospital, "The allure of souping continues to grow....Not only do the herbs and spices have a host of health benefits, but the vegetable pulp contains fiber which can increase our sense of satiety."[1]

SOUPING VERSUS JUICING

I'm known as the Juice Lady. I've been juicing for decades and teaching people about the healing power of fresh juice. I'm not convinced that souping is better than juicing because nothing is quite the same as live, raw juice. That being said, juicing does have strong benefits, including less mess and less fuss and more fiber than juicing. It also can be more satisfying than juicing. Juicing is to extract the juice from the fiber. Raw blended soups retain all the fiber from vegetables; they are the whole food blended up. Souping also includes making gently warmed, cooked soups and the more traditional long-simmered soups. In the winter when it's hard to drink just juice for a short cleanse, warm soup can be a lifesaver. And many people need something more substantial than just clear juice when they fast or do a cleanse.

Actually, any time of year soups, including blended soups and smoothies, can be combined with juice to make a healthy and satisfying menu plan.

People love the idea of making raw soup because it is so easy—just chop, drop your ingredients in the blender, and go. Such raw soups are the ultimate on-the-go meal. Take your blended soup with you to drink on your commute. Keep some in the freezer for a busy night. Make them healthy with organic ingredients and the freshest produce available to get the most health benefits possible. Making your own soup helps you avoid preservatives, bad fats, BPA (sometimes found in canned soups), and sugar.

You can sip your way to a slimmer you because soup is filling and nourishing. It satisfies—whether it's a cold, raw soup or a hot soup. Soup is a way to pump up your metabolism and keep fit. And it is excellent for the immune system, helping you prevent colds and flu.

I'm about to show you how this ultimate comfort food can help you lose weight, detoxify your system, and heal your body. Soon you will be blending up yummy, raw soups and simmering pots of comforting aromatic soup. Grab your stockpot and blender. It's time to make soup!

CHAPTER 1

MY OWN JOURNEY
TO HEALTH

*Those who think they have no
time for healthy eating will sooner or
later have to find time for illness.*[1]
—EDWARD STANLEY, EARL OF DERBY

WHEN I THINK about soup, the first word that
comes to my mind is *comfort*. How many times
have you needed a comforting, soothing bowl of soup
when you were sick? Like you, I've had my bouts with
upper respiratory infections and flu. When I was a child,
chicken soup with lots of vegetables and garlic was always
my grandmother's remedy for such illnesses. It is a part
of my healing regimen to this day.

But I've had more serious challenges as an adult, times
when I needed a huge bowl of comfort that included but
reached far beyond a bowl of soup. I share my stories
with you to give you hope that you can overcome whatever challenges you face. This is chicken soup for your soul.

SICK AND TIRED OF
BEING SICK AND TIRED

My health journey began after I had been sick for a few years and just kept getting worse. In fact, I was so sick and tired I could barely walk around the house. I wondered, "Will I ever be well again?" I eventually had to quit my job because of chronic fatigue syndrome and fibromyalgia. They made me so sick I was unable work. I felt as though I had a never-ending flu. Constantly feverish with swollen glands and perennial lethargy, I was in constant pain. My body ached all over.

I moved back to my father's home in Colorado to try to recover, but not one doctor had a recommendation for what I should do to facilitate healing. So I went to some health-food stores and browsed while talking with some employees, and I read a few books. I decided that everything I'd been doing—eating fast food, having granola for dinner, and not eating vegetables—was tearing down my health rather than healing my body.

I read about juicing and whole foods, and it made sense to me. I bought a juicer and designed a program I could follow. I kicked off my new program with a five-day juice fast. On the fifth day my body expelled a tumor the size of a golf ball with blue blood vessels attached. I was surprised and actually encouraged. I thought I'd be well in short order. But that was not to be the case.

I continued juicing and ate a nearly perfect diet of live and whole foods for three months. There were ups and downs throughout. Some days I felt encouraged that I was making some progress, but other days I felt worse. The days I took a step back were discouraging and made me wonder if health was my elusive dream. No one told me about detox reactions, which was what I was experiencing. I was obviously very toxic, and my body was cleansing away all that stuff that had made me sick. This caused the not-so-good days in the midst of the promising ones.

But one day I woke up early—around 8:00 a.m., which was early for me—without an alarm. I felt as if someone had given me a new body during the night. I had so much energy I actually wanted to go jogging! What had happened? This new sensation of health seemed to have appeared with the morning sun, but my body had been healing all along; the healing simply had not manifested until that day. What a wonderful sense of being alive! I looked and felt completely renewed. With my juicer in tow and a new lifestyle fully embraced, I returned to Southern California a few weeks later to finish writing my first book. For nearly a year I enjoyed great health and more energy and stamina than I had ever had before.

But just ahead was a shattering event.

DEATH KNOCKED ON MY DOOR

It all started one Fourth of July in Southern California. I was single, house-sitting for some friends of our family, and working at a restaurant so I could pay my way through school that fall. The house-sitting job didn't pay very much, but every little bit helped. I'd spent the day with friends at a backyard barbecue and watched fireworks from their patio. I returned to the home I was caring for a little before midnight and went straight to bed. I was awakened at 3:00 a.m. shivering. The home was just four miles from the ocean, so the night air was always cool, even in the summer. But that night I was unusually cold. I pulled the covers up and then noticed that the door to the patio was wide open. "How did that happen?" I wondered. I'd made sure it was locked when I went to bed. I was just about to get up and close it, when I noticed him—a young guy in shorts and no shirt crouched in the corner of the room.

I went into panic mode—and denial. "This can't be happening," I thought. But before I had any further chance to think or act, the perpetrator sprang into action. He had a pipe tucked in his shorts, and it became his weapon. He began beating me over the head and yelling, "Now you are dead!" The pounding reverberated through my body and soul. We struggled until we rolled off the bed and the pipe flew out of his hands. I heard him open the desk drawer above my head searching for a weapon, I assume, but he found none (although the detective saw his blood smeared prints stopped just centimeters short of a hunting knife). That's when the man attempted to strangle me. I felt my spirit leave my body. In my mind I said, "Father, receive me into Your hands." I felt my spirit leave; it seemed as if I was traveling at the speed of light.

Then suddenly I was outside at the end of the dog run, clinging to the fence and screaming for help.

On my third scream, when I was about to pass out again, a neighbor heard my cry for help. By 4:00 a.m. I was lying on a cold gurney in the hospital with a police officer seated nearby trying to get some answers while nurses tried to assess the damage. I could see the horrors of what happened to my right hand. It was split wide open. I could see deep inside. My ring finger hung by a small piece of skin. They shaved the top of my head and a nurse said she was drawing a road map of my head injuries. Then I was wheeled off to surgery.

The top hand surgeon of Orange County just happened to be at the hospital that morning. Hours later I got the bad news. The surgeon was the best, and he did the best he could, but two of my knuckles had been reduced to mostly bone fragments and powder. He put three metal pins in my hand to hold it together, sewed my finger back on, and sewed my hand up. There was little hope that I would ever be able to use it again. As a writer working on my first book, that was about the worst news I could get.

NIGHTMARES AND THE ANGEL IN THE MORNING

Months after the surgery my hand surgeon said there was nothing he could do for me. My hand wasn't healing. It was in such bad shape he couldn't even put in plastic knuckles. He gave me no hope that I could ever use my hand again. I talked to God that evening through my tears. I asked if He could just let me know what His plans were for my hand, for me. I'd accept that, but I needed to know where I stood and what the future held. An angel showed up in my room—at five o'clock in the morning the next day. The angel said, "You will be completely healed!" My removable cast was off and I was moving my fingers like nothing had happened. Then the angel told me my hand would go back to its injured state, but I would get progressively better until my hand would be completely whole. That was the sweetest voice I've ever heard. And it all came true.

After returning home from the hospital after the attack, I couldn't sleep one wink at night. Terror struck my soul and wouldn't let go. Nights were torturous. My eyes would sting when I'd try to read. I would have five lights on in my room all night. I was exhausted, but there was no way I could relax enough to sleep. I never knew how long and lonely a night could be until I couldn't sleep. I could sleep only a few hours when the sun came up, and my sleep was disturbed with nightmares. I was so exhausted I could barely move.

I was suffering from PTSD, but no one talked about that then. Nevertheless, I had many of the symptoms—nightmares, flashbacks, triggers, and feeling like the world was a dangerous place. I had trouble concentrating. I was often startled by loud noises, and I was terrified to be alone. I learned from a support group for victims of violent crimes that many victims commit suicide because they just can't deal with the symptoms following their trauma.

But I chose to survive. Bit by bit I healed enough to sleep at night. Several years after the attack, when I would travel—mostly to QVC to represent the George Foreman Grills on air—I was fearful at night alone in my hotel room. I would go through an elaborate ritual of stacking furniture up in front of the door, moving whatever was movable and topping it off with a wastebasket. I felt that if someone tried to get in, everything would fall and it would wake me up, along with a few other people. This would give me time to call hotel security for help. This ritual was exhausting and very abnormal. I prayed a lot for peace and safety. Gradually I no longer needed to stack up furniture, and a feeling of being safe in the world returned.

HEALING WOUNDS

The worst part of my injuries was my inner pain. All the emotional pain of the attack hooked up with the pain and trauma of my past and rushed in like an emotional tsunami. My childhood was riddled with loss, trauma, and anxiety. My brother died when I was two. My mother died of cancer when I was six. I can't remember much about her death—the memories seemed blocked—but my cousin said I fainted at her funeral. That told me a lot.

I lived for the next three years with my father and maternal grandparents, but Grandpa John, the love of my life, died when I was nine. I felt as if I couldn't breathe for days. Four years later my father was involved in a very tragic situation that would take far too long to discuss here. He was no longer in my daily life. I was terrified about my future. My grandmother was eighty-six, and I had no idea how many more years she would live. The next year I moved to Oregon to live with an aunt and uncle until I graduated from high school.

Wrapped in my soul was a big package of anguish, fear, and pain with all sorts of triggers, and the attack only made this worse. After the attack, when I was just about ready to give up, I met three ladies that I call my "kitchen angels." They prayed for me week after week around their kitchen table. I began the slow, long journey of recovery in body and soul. To heal physically, mentally, and emotionally took every ounce of my will, faith, and trust in God.

I did deep spiritual work, sought alternative medical help, took extra vitamins and minerals, resumed vegetable juicing, and experienced the emotional release of healing prayer and numerous detox programs. I met a nutritionally minded physician who had healed his own slow-mending broken bones with lots of vitamin-mineral IVs. He gave me similar IVs. This, along with juicing, cleansing, fasting, nutritional supplements, a nearly perfect diet, prayer, and physical therapy, helped my bones and other injuries to heal.

After I followed this regimen for a number of months, what my hand surgeon said was impossible became a reality—I had a fully restored, fully functional hand.

The surgeon told me it wasn't possible to put in plastic knuckles because of the hand's poor condition and that I'd never use my right hand again. But what the angel told me at five o'clock in the morning came true. My knuckles did indeed re-form out of powder and bone fragments, and the function of my hand returned. A day came when my doctor told me I was completely healed, and though he admitted he didn't believe in miracles, he said, "You're the closest thing I've seen to one." The healing of my hand was indeed a miracle! I had a useful right hand again, and my career in writing was not over, as I had feared it would be.

Before my hand was healed, I also experienced so much pain in my neck that my doctor wanted to fuse it. I refused that option, choosing to trust God. After I was healed, the pain was gone and I was able to turn my neck with complete range of motion. I had no more symptoms. The miraculous part of this story remains that an X-ray several years ago still showed I had two crushed discs in my neck. I encourage you to trust God no matter how bad the report regarding your health or life's situation. Circumstances may look really bleak, but trust in God.

Though my inner wounds were more severe than the physical injuries and were harder to heal, they mended too. I experienced healing from the painful memories and trauma of the attack and the wounds from the past through prayer, letting go, forgiveness, laying on of hands, and deep emotional healing work. I cried endless buckets of tears that had been pent up in my soul and found release. Forgiveness and letting go came in stages and proved to be an integral part of my total healing. I had to be honest about what I really felt and to be willing to face the pain and toxic emotions confined inside and then let them go.

Finally, after a very long journey, I felt free. Eventually I could even celebrate the Fourth of July without fear. Today that day is like any other holiday.

A SLEEP CRISIS REVISITED

Suddenly in 2017 I found myself grasping at anything for hope, anything for help.

February 2 rode in on a dark horse. My husband startled me at 2:30 a.m. He didn't mean to, but when he woke me up, my whole body went into a state of panic. It seemed to be some kind of flashback to the night of the attack and a revisit of PTSD I experienced afterward. Preparing my body to run from the proverbial lion on the loose, adrenaline, norepinephrine, and cortisol pumped through my veins like a shot of uppers. I didn't go back to sleep the rest of the night, and the next night when I woke up around the same time, the same thing happened. So it continued for more than two weeks. I'd wake up between 1:30 a.m. and 3:00 a.m. and be too afraid to go back to sleep. All the fight-or-flight hormones would start pumping out, and nothing could override them to get me back to sleep. Panic is the devil of the nighttime.

I tried everything to get over this. I called my

naturopathic doctor and got some herbal remedies. I ordered an anti-anxiety herbal blend. I tried amino acids and Chinese herbal teas. I ate protein at night for night-time hypoglycemia. I took a variety of supplements for my stressed-out adrenals. I talked with various holistic practitioners and bought every remedy they suggested. I tried a natural muscle relaxant. I bought a bevy of stuff from the health-food store, including lavender oil. I lay on a BioMat and got a massage. I even tried a friend's sleeping pills. I retested with the Brain Neurotransmitter testing and changed up my amino acids. Nothing, absolutely nothing, worked. Don't get me wrong. All these remedies and interventions are helpful for many people, but no matter what I tried, I was back in full-blown anxiety when night time rolled around, just as I had experienced years ago, just after the attack. Some nights I didn't sleep one minute. It was brutal, and I didn't even feel human. I was trying to write this book, but it was nearly impossible.

As my husband looked at all the supplements I had assembled on our counter to try and help my exhausted, sleep-deprived body, he said I was like the woman we're told about in Luke 8:43–48. This woman had a bleeding condition that had dogged her for twelve years. She had spent all her money on doctors and treatments that didn't help. In fact, she steadily grew worse. And to make matters even more desperate, she was considered "unclean" by Jewish law because of her bleeding condition. That meant she couldn't enter the temple for worship. And anyone or anything she touched would be considered unclean, so she was an outcast in her own community. That meant that when she touched Jesus, He was unclean. But she was so desperate she pushed through the crowd believing that if she could touch just His robe, she would be healed. And the second she touched His clothes, her bleeding stopped.

Though I had been praying for help all along, I had been trying to figure it out on my own with holistic doctors and remedies. When I finally did what the woman who touched Jesus's robe did, my situation turned around. It was Sunday, February 19. I'd exhausted everything I knew to do. That's when I surrendered it all. I couldn't do it, and I needed help far beyond what any doctor or remedy could offer me. That was the night I touched Jesus's robe. I felt the stress dissipate. It was like a bird flew out the window. I fell asleep at 9:30 p.m. and didn't wake up until 5:30 a.m. And then I went back to sleep.

Though it was ultimately Jesus who healed me after my desperate cry for help, there were some techniques and treatments that helped me, as well. One thing that helped a great deal were relaxation techniques my husband (who is a psychotherapist) taught me with the emWave machine from HeartMath. I learned breathing techniques and how to clear my mind of stressful thoughts. Through this product, I played (and enjoyed playing!) a gold coin game on the computer that measured how often I stayed in a relaxation zone. I now make sure I take several breathing breaks throughout the day. It's a great help when it comes to relaxing sleep at night.

My adrenals also did need healing and help. They were stressed long before the incident on February 2. We moved three times in a year and a half, and I had written two books in that time. And someone made some soups for us, and unbeknownst to us, had put a lot of sugar in them. My adrenal glands are very sensitive to sugar; it essentially gets them stuck on, pumping out stress hormones to my body as if a bear is chasing me. I never eat sugar, so when I accidentally did, I had to follow my own advice in my book *The Juice Lady's Remedies for Stress and Adrenal Fatigue*. I had to watch my diet strictly.

The brain neurotransmitter test and the recommended amino acid supplements also helped me a great deal. The test show my serotonin and GABA were too high—a sign that my body was over-excreting these substances to bring down my excitatory neurotransmitters. As the practitioner explained, eventually my body would wear out from overproduction and start producing less. The amino acid supplementation tailored to my specific needs helped a great deal.

All these steps were my part of my healing, but the big part was God's.

Part of God's healing was a prayer of release, which helped me immensely. Finally I could lie down in peace and experience Proverbs 3:24: "When you lie down, you will not be afraid; yes, you will lie down and your sleep will be sweet." This prayer may be helpful for you as well.

Father God, I choose by an act of my will to loose from my soul all fear, worry, anxiety, abuse, trauma, witchcraft, greed, poverty, lack, lies, and accusations. I loose all critical, judgmental words spoken to me or by me. I loose from my soul all images, sounds, and words that would in any way disturb my soul. I loose from my soul all violence that I've watched, read about, or experienced. I loose from my soul all hate, viciousness, revenge, and anger. I loose all addictions. I loose anything that steals my peace or steals my destiny. I loose anything that crushes me or steals from me. I loose it all from my soul in Jesus's name.

Now, Father, I bind to my soul Your love, Your life, Your presence, Your peace, Your creativity, Your sound wisdom, Your discernment, Your understanding, Your joy, Your celebration, Your relaxation, and Your laughter. I thank You, Father, that my soul can prosper and be in health because it is now whole.

I've always said I'm the lab rat for the world. Through my struggles, others have found great hope. I pray this last struggle wasn't in vain. I pray it offers you some rays of hope and some useful tips for whatever you may be going through. This is soup for your soul. Now let's turn to soup for your body.

CHAPTER 2

SOUP: THE ULTIMATE COMFORT FOOD

Good broth will resurrect the dead.
—SOUTH AMERICAN PROVERB

I HAVE FOND MEMORIES of eating a bowl of my grandmother's steaming potato soup on cold winter nights. Whether it's a warm bowl of soup on a cold evening or a refreshing cup of chilled, raw soup when the weather is warm, soup is comforting, nourishing, and healthy. I love the aromas that fill the house as a pot of hot soup simmers in my kitchen. It brings back many memories of childhood. I lived with my grandmother after my mother died when I was six. She was a great soup maker. Two of her best recipes were her potato and corn chowder and her chicken noodle soup.

I've carried on her tradition and make soup often. It can really hit the spot almost any time. I'm excited about this book about soup because making your own delicious homemade brew is a far healthier choice than any canned version. Homemade soup is BPA free and has no preservatives or fillers, and is not high sodium. In fact, you can make sure you use only healthy sea salt or pink Himalayan salt, organic vegetables, and other healthy ingredients. You can make your soup gluten-free, dairy-free, sugar-free, and soy-free, which is what all the recipes are in this book.

Soup is one of the easiest meals you can prepare. That's probably one reason why it's making a big comeback today. Plus, your efforts can pay off for days. The soup you make today could be dinner tonight and lunch tomorrow, but it can also be frozen for the future when you need something fast. I like to freeze batches of soup in plastic bags or glass bowls. (Before freezing, let the soup chill overnight in the refrigerator. When you are ready to eat the soup, take it out of the freezer in the morning and let it thaw in the refrigerator. By evening it is ready to be warmed up.) It's nice to have frozen soup on hand when a friend gets sick or your neighbor has had oral surgery and can't eat anything. Blended soup is the perfect answer. In fact, I recently blended a borscht soup for our neighbor.

SOUP AND SOCIETY

Soup is older than you may think. There is evidence that human beings started making soup thousands of years ago. Its current popularity has been aided by steady advances in technology, from the invention of pottery to modern kitchenware. Since the nineteenth century, technology and increased food supplies have contributed to modern methods of preparing soups. As a result, increasing numbers of people, both the rich and the very poor, have come to depend on soup.

Did you know that the modern
restaurant industry first
evolved around establishments
that served only soup?[1]

Because soup has evolved with society itself, soups are deeply rooted in local traditions and microcultures. Accordingly a bowl of soup is a great way to connect with a region. Almost every popular form of soup has a rich history rooted in local tradition and the history behind it. You can enhance your eating experience by taking time to understand the cultures behind the different soups you consume. For example, soup often offers insight into the climate and weather patterns of a region. Many warmer countries have a tradition of serving cold soups for starters and desserts.

GO FORTH AND MAKE SOUP!

The United States soup market is currently experiencing a period of growth that is expected to continue into the immediate future. Why are so many people jumping on the soup bandwagon? Here are six reasons:

1. **Soups are economical**. Many meals are expensive, but it is not so with soup. Nearly all the standard soups are inexpensive if you make them yourself, using basic ingredients. Many people have grown up with parents who worked hard to support their families; soup is often used as a staple to feed families in such situations.

2. **Soups are easily digested**. The way soups are prepared make them highly digestible, giving you more bang for your buck. (This is also a reason why soups are excellent for weight loss, the subject of chapter 5.)

3. **Soups are easy to make**. You don't need to be a culinary genius or have special kitchen equipment to make soup. All standard soups are easy to make and require only basic kitchen supplies.

4. **Soups are nutritious**. Unlike many healthy meals that offer only one or two aspects of the nutrition you need (protein, fiber, whole grains), most soups give a complete nutritional balance. Moreover, soups can be easily customized to your dietary needs by simply adding what you require and omitting or exchanging what

foods you cannot have or need to limit. Soups are also an effective way to ingest medicinal spices and herbs.

5. **Soups save time**. Let's face it—most of us lead incredibly busy lives. It can be challenging to find the time to cook. You can save much time by making a large batch of soup and freezing some of it or even just refrigerating it for the next day. Unlike other meals that go off quickly, soups retain their flavor even after being frozen.

6. **Soups satisfy the appetite without adding lots of calories**. Research shows that soup helps satisfy hunger cravings without adding additional calories. In many cases soup is more satisfying than eating solid food.

Tip! If you are making an entire meal out of soup, be sure to choose a soup that includes protein. Did you know that lentils and beans are among the best, and cheapest, sources of protein available?

WHY SOUP IS
GOOD FOR YOU

We all know we need vegetables in our diet, but often, no matter hard we try, it seems as if we always fall short of the recommended daily amount of vegetables. Soup is a simple solution to this problem. Incorporating regular bowls of soup into your diet helps you increase your vegetable intake, and it helps you enjoy those vegetables.

Soups are also good for you because they enable you to lose weight and stay healthy at the same time. Many people who try to lose weight do so at the expense of nutrients. Soup is a great way to shed unwanted pounds *without* sacrificing nutrients.

Stock, Broth, and Soup

"In general, broth is a liquid made by boiling meat, bones, or vegetables. There are many types of broths, based on what is being cooked. For example, Bieler Broth, a vegetable broth made with green beans, zucchini, and celery is a supportive remedy used in detoxification or cleansing protocols. Consommé, a rich broth made from meat, is another example. It is prepared by reducing, or prolonged simmering. Stock is another word used synonymously with broth, though some chefs denote stock as being made from bones whereas broth is made from meat....Soup is a similar term referring to simmered vegetables, meat, and seasonings, and is defined by *Random House Webster's Dictionary* as a liquid food. The difference is that soup contains solids such as meat, beans, grains or vegetables (sometimes disguised by a purée) while a broth is the liquid in which solids have been simmered and then discarded. Soup is what we think of as having for a meal. Broth is a starting ingredient for soup or something we sip alone, and must be prepared separately beforehand."[2]

SOUP RULES: TIPS FOR MAKING THE BEST SOUP EVER!

If you google tips on how to make soup, you may quickly find yourself saturated in an overwhelming amount of information. To keep things simple, I have distilled advice on soup preparation down to the following steps.

- **Double the quantity**. If you make a big batch of soup in the beginning of the week, it can serve your needs for many days. Soups can easily be doubled or even tripled with hardly any additional work. Moreover, soups keep well in the refrigerator or freezer without losing their tastiness. Some soups even taste *better* after three or four days in the fridge as the flavors mature.

- **Get the most out of your vegetables**. There is a reason vegetables such as onion, garlic, celery, and carrots are popular in soups. These aromatic vegetables add a fullness of flavor to the entire soup. To get the most out of these flavors, sauté the vegetables in coconut or olive oil to soften them before adding other ingredients.

- **Stagger the cook time**. Different vegetables require varying lengths of time to soften. For example, a parsnip will take much longer to soften than cabbage. Stagger when you add the ingredients so all the vegetables can finish cooking at around the same time.

- **Don't overcomplicate the process**. Sometimes recipe books can overcomplicate the process of soup preparation. Although soups come in many different shapes and sizes, there are four basic stages to preparing a good soup. First, sauté your aromatic vegetables. Second, add stock, broth, or water along with the other ingredients. Third, bring ingredients to boil. Fourth, turn down the heat to simmer (this is crucial to avoid the vegetables becoming mushy).

- **Don't over-season**. Americans typically prefer highly seasoned food—usually including lots of salt. By all means, add salt and pepper to your soup, but preferably at the end and only a little. Also go easy on heavily seasoned stocks. Learn to taste the subtle flavors of the vegetables and herbs; your soup will not only be healthier for you, but you'll also begin enjoying it more.

- **Take stock of your stock**. If your goal is to produce soup with a good flavor, it all hinges on the quality of your stock. A stock that is badly flavored will spoil the entire pot of soup. You can also make a delicious stock yourself by boiling bones and leftover pieces of meat. When boiling bones, add a little apple cider vinegar to help draw out the minerals hidden inside the bones. (For further information on this, see the section on bone marrow broth below.) Homemade stock is always preferable, but if you're after something quick, most health food stores provide nutritious and healthy stock powder you can add to your soup. Make sure to read the ingredients first to make sure the stock powder is completely natural.

- **Know how to thicken**. To thicken soup, blend part or all of the soup, blend cashews or rice with some of the soup, or use a plant milk with arrowroot blended with the soup. (By the way, cashews or cashew butter add a creamy taste to the soup without dairy.)

- **Don't be afraid to use leftovers**. Don't be afraid to be adventurous and incorporate ingredients you need to use, even if they aren't called for by the actual recipe. Louis P. DeGouy observed that "from time immemorial, soups and broths have been the worldwide medium for utilizing what we call the kitchen by-products, or as the French call them, the '*desertes de la table*' (leftovers)."[3]

MOST POPULAR SOUPS

It's easy to get stuck in a rut with home cooking, rotating between the same few, familiar dishes. Sometimes it can be helpful to break out of the box to see what other people are making. To help you be adventurous, here is a list of some of the most popular soups in America right now. Each of these soups is popular for a reason—they taste delicious.

- **Clam chowder soup**: This soup was introduced to New England by settlers and has become a favorite throughout all of the United States. Technically any soup that contains both clams and broth qualifies as a clam chowder. This soup is very versatile, working well with a variety of other ingredients including diced potatoes, onions, and celery. Some people prefer a thick creamy base, which can be made with plant milk as well as dairy, others prefer a red broth (from fresh tomatoes), and still other people prefer a clear broth of clam juice.

- **Chicken noodle soup**: In Asia noodles have been used in soups for hundreds of years, if not more. In the eighteenth century Italians used noodle soup as a convenient food for sick people because it was easy to digest. Noodle soup made its way to America, where it became a popular convenience food in the twentieth century. It was not until the 1930s, however, that noodle soup was combined with the already popular chicken soup. In 1934 Campbell's company brought out "Noodle with Chicken Soup." Years later a radio host accidentally referred to this as "Chicken Noodle Soup." Thinking it was a new type of soup, people began flocking to the stores to find "Chicken Noodle Soup." Campbell eventually changed the name on the packaging, and the rest is history.[4]

- **French onion soup**: People have been eating onion soups since as far back as Roman times. Our modern variation originates from eighteenth-century France, where it was produced using beef broth and caramelized onions.[5] The main ingredients are onions, beef or chicken stock, croutons, and grated cheese. It is often used as a starter and always appears on the menu at full-service restaurants.

- **Tortilla soup**: Tortilla soup is one of the most exciting dishes, made increasingly popular by America's growing Latino population. Of Mexican origin, this soup consists of broth (chicken or vegetable) with roasted tomatoes, onion, garlic, chilies, and tortillas (beans are also sometimes used). The tortillas, from which the soup derives its name, are cut into strips and fried before being added to the soup.

- **Vegetable soup**: Along with meat soups, vegetable soups have their roots in ancient history. The Spartans were known for eating a vegetable soup known as "black broth."[6] One of the reasons for the popularity of this soup is its versatility. With a good stock and the correct cooking method, it's hard to go wrong with vegetable soup, no matter what vegetables you incorporate into it.

- **Minestrone soup**: This popular Italian soup consists of seasonal vegetables cooked in a broth (usually a bean broth), often with the addition of pasta or rice. Since there is no fixed recipe for this soup, it can vary from place to place and from season to season. This soup may have originated with Latin tribes in the area that later became part of the Roman Empire.

- **Chicken soup**: Although the origins of chicken soup remain shrouded in mystery, it has been a popular folk remedy for colds as far back as the twelfth century, if not earlier. Most of the countries in the world have their own special variation of chicken soup, which usually consists of a base of chicken broth with added root vegetables and herbs.

- **Lobster bisque**: Lobster bisque, once a gourmet food only found at high-end restaurants, is now becoming popular in the mainstream. Of French origin, it incorporates puréed lobster into a creamy and highly seasoned broth. Some variations have added chunks of lobster to the bisque.

TYPES OF SOUPS

Soups can be categorized according to the following three basic types:

1. **Hot soups**: The soups that most people in America are familiar with are hot; the popular soups mentioned in the above list are all hot soups. But this is actually only one of three different types of soups.

2. **Cold soups**: Cold soups come in many forms, both sweet and savory. The most popular type of cold soup is gazpacho, a chilled vegetable-based soup of Spanish origin. There are many other types of cold soups, ranging from yogurt soups to rich and creamy dessert soups.

3. **Raw soups**: There are as many recipes for raw soups as there are for hot soups. Raw soups can be served cold as a variation on green smoothies or slowly warmed up (but not brought over a temperature of 118 degrees—so they remain raw). Many people are skeptical of raw soups until they try them and taste how delicious they can be.

BONE BROTH WITH MARROW

Bone broth can become the base of a soup or be consumed by itself. It is made with bone marrow, a fatty, nutrient-dense substance found in the central cavity of the bone. It helps manufacture of cells in the blood and contains collagen protein fibers, one of the key building blocks of the body. Consuming bone marrow has been linked to a variety of health benefits:[7]

- Improved brain function

- Healthy bones

- Immune system support

- Healing after injury or fracture

These benefits will be discussed in-depth later in the book. To harvest the marrow, simply simmer bones in water with a little apple cider vinegar. You can add a variety of vegetables and herbs for a richer broth. (See chapter 8 for my bone broth recipe.)

SOUP FOR YOUR SOUL

As Amanda drove the final stretch of the road to her grandmother's house, she reflected on how little everything had changed since her childhood. The same forest of paper birch rustled gently in the wind, giving the woodland a delicate and magical atmosphere.

Amanda's parents moved frequently when she was a child. The nomadic lifestyle meant that Amanda's childhood was far from stable. It seemed that as soon as she settled into a new school and began making friends, the family would uproot themselves and start over again somewhere else.

The one constant in Amanda's life was the yearly visit to her grandmother. Every New Year's Eve, without exception, the family would pile in the car and make the drive to her house, where they would stay for two weeks.

Amanda has always found it comforting to know that, whatever problems she might be facing in her life, the yearly visit to Grandma would happen without fail.

There had always been plenty to do there. Amanda enjoyed making forts in the woods with her cousins. Before he died, her grandfather would sometimes take the children on expeditions to spy on animals in the woods. When it snowed, Amanda would go out with her cousins to build snowmen or go sledding down the hill behind the house. When they got so cold they couldn't stand it anymore, they would pile into the house where her grandmother would serve them her delicious chicken soup.

Of all the things Amanda missed, it was probably the chicken soup she missed most of all. The comforting flavors, the unique combination of aromatic herbs and spices—these always seemed to reassure Amanda that everything would be OK. After all, as Laurie Colwin wrote, "To feel safe and warm on a cold wet night, all you really need is soup."[8]

If ever Amanda was troubled, Grandma seemed to

know it. Without saying anything, she would quietly bring Amanda a steaming bowl of her soup. Just the aroma of the parsley and thyme in the soup seemed to have a calming effect on Amanda's soul. As Amanda sipped the soup, Grandma would often sit with her. They didn't need to say anything—just being together made everything all right.

Grandma said she had learned to make the soup from her mother, who had learned from her mother, who had learned it from her mother. Once or twice Amanda had tried to make the soup herself, but somehow it never tasted the same. Grandma always used root vegetables from her own garden in the soup, which probably had something to do with the wholesome, comforting, and delicious flavor.

After her grandfather died, the family had tried to persuade her grandmother to move into the city, but she had always insisted on staying in the woods. Although this frustrated the rest of the family, Amanda was secretly glad; she couldn't imagine Grandma living anywhere else.

Amanda's visits stopped the year she went off to college. At first, life in the big city had been exciting. There had been so much to see, learn, and do. Amanda made new friends and quickly forgot about her trips to her grandmother's home. During her freshman year she had tried to write to Grandma every week, but eventually she fell out of the habit, distracted by so much other activity.

In her senior year Amanda hit a rough patch. She wasn't exactly depressed, but she was disillusioned about the direction her life was heading. As Amanda wrestled with the problems she was facing, she realized that the things that meant the most to her were the little things she had taken for granted: the yearly visits to Grandma's house, playing with her cousins in the woods, and especially coming in from the cold to a bowl of grandmother's steaming chicken soup.

All this flashed through Amanda's mind as she drove along the winding lane. It had only been last week that she made the spur-of-the-moment decision to drive to Grandma's on New Year's break. She had written to tell Grandma she would be visiting but hadn't had time to wait for a reply (Grandmother didn't have a phone or e-mail).

As Amanda approached the final stretch of road, she suddenly was plagued with doubts. Hesitating, she decided to park the car and walk the rest of the way up the long driveway in order to collect her thoughts.

She had changed so much during the last three years, and not all for the better. What would Grandma think of her now? Would Grandma resent the fact that she had stopped writing letters three years ago? Did Grandma even get her letter saying she was coming?

Worst of all was the fear that maybe Grandma had changed. She was much older now, and people said she was beginning to lose her memory.

As Amanda approached the house, a wintry breeze began to blow. Soon soft snowflakes were falling, gently tickling her nose. Through the wind and snow, Amanda thought she detected a familiar smell. It was the smell of Grandmother's chicken soup!

Suddenly the door swung open and there stood Grandma, a beaming smile on her face.

"Oh, Amanda dear—I am so happy to see you!" she said, holding her arms out in embrace.

Tears welled in Amanda's eyes as they stood in the doorway and hugged.

"But do come in, come in out of the cold," Grandmother said. "I knew you would be famished after the long drive, so I made some of your favorite chicken soup."

Amanda went in, quietly shutting the door behind her.

Amanda's story encapsulates an important point about soup—soup is not simply good for the body; it is also good for the soul. Throughout the years many have agreed, including Louis De Gouy, author of *The Soup Book*:[9]

> Soup is cuisine's kindest course. It breathes reassurance; it steams consolation; after a weary day it promotes sociability, as the five o'clock cup of tea or the cocktail hour.

Different soups bring back memories, sometimes evoking forgotten associations. I have memories of my mother-in-law's minestrone soup. She made it often for all of us. Many times when my husband and I stopped by, cold and hungry, she had a big pot of minestrone soup on the stove. I miss her soup; it has been years since she made it.

The slow method by which soup is naturally consumed

makes it the perfect dish for facilitating connection with others. A bowl of soup invites us to connect with friends and family, to slow down from our fast-paced lives and be centered in the presence of those we love. Through soup we can reconnect with the things that mean the most to us.

CHAPTER 3

LIVING FOODS: THE ESSENTIAL FOUNDATION

*People who love to eat are
always the best people.*[1]

—JULIA CHILD

WHAT IF I told you there's something you could do
that would greatly improve your health, help you
look younger, and give your skin a healthy glow that's
more attractive than a tan? Interested?

Eat living foods!

So what are living foods anyway? They are foods that
are alive rather than overly cooked, which would destroy
the vitamins, enzymes, and biophotons. These foods
give us life! That's what souping is all about—providing
a delicious way to consume foods that truly feed your
body. You'll get all this goodness in the delicious raw
soup and gently warmed soup recipes in chapter 8. If you
keep the temperature of a soup at 118 degrees or below, it

is considered a raw soup. But even the soups that simmer all day have health benefits.

THE ABUNDANT LIFESTYLE

Do you ever feel as if you're living a suboptimal existence? Maybe you suffer from lack of energy, depression, poor memory, frequent colds and flu, poor sleep, lack of joy in your life, sore muscles, pain, headaches, or a general malaise and a feeling that things just aren't quite right. Your birthright is abundant health and the joyous living it brings. With a lifestyle that includes plenty of raw foods, you can take a step toward this lifestyle each day.

Why not begin today the transition to the living foods lifestyle with fabulous homemade soups so you can live the life you long for. Even if you just make half of your diet raw, you've made a great improvement. So many of the raw-food programs I've looked at were all or nothing. You either go all raw or forget it. Many people feel very discouraged when they think about trying to go to a raw-food diet. They feel they just can't do it. However, if you know you have some grace, that you can add raw food to your diet one soup or salad at a time, it may be easier. You may find hope in the fact that you can feel better with each and every small step, such as eating raw soups.

People often ask me what a living foods day looks like. To eat a living-food diet, start each day with something alive, something such as a blended raw soup or smoothie. You could have another raw soup or even juice in the afternoon as a pick-me-up. Have a salad for lunch or dinner, and munch on some veggie sticks for a snack; I often have baby carrots and fresh green peas in the refrigerator for this purpose. For dessert you could eat a serving of low-sugar fruit. If you strive to make half your diet living food, you will be taking great strides toward the abundant lifestyle. If you have been struggling with your health, you could add in an extra raw soup or some fresh juice. If you have digestive problems, you could do a one- to three-day juice fast to give your system a rest before moving into this diet. (See my book *The Juice Lady's Guide to Fasting*).

I have observed that on days when I eat mainly cooked foods, I'm hungrier and don't feel quite satisfied. Maybe you too have noticed that by the end of a day eating cooked foods, you're still hungry. This is why raw soups, green smoothies, and fresh juice are so amazing. They satisfy the body because they are loaded with nutrients. This, along with getting rid of yeast and parasites, is a big answer to cravings. And don't forget to get your stress under control too. Stress can almost make you want to eat the wallpaper right off your wall! All of these tips are part of the abundant lifestyle.

I've heard from people all over the world who say their health and energy really improved when they increased their raw-food consumption. This was true for me too; years ago I had chronic fatigue syndrome. I was so tired I could barely walk around the house. But gradually I gained energy by increasing my consumption of raw foods. Raw and blended soups are packed with nutrients that enliven the body, such as biophotons, which are light rays of energy that plants get from the sun. When you cook food, you lose that energy. That's why some people call cooked food "dead food." The larger the light stores in the food, the better it is for your body. That's why sun-ripened and fresh picked vegetables are ideal. Then these little light rays can get into your cells and spark them up.[2]

If you begin to eat more live foods than you do cooked foods, you will see a change in your whole biochemistry. Because live foods give you the best nutrition, you'll find you aren't as hungry and need fewer calories. It's a little bit like getting a reboot for your computer and it runs so much faster.

Are you feeling a little lighter or a bit more energized just thinking about this? That's my prayer for you—that you can experience the abundant lifestyle and the restful sleep it brings with it; that you can be energized and get a jump start for your creativity; that you no longer experience foggy brain because biophotons electrically stimulate the brain; that your immune system would get stronger and you'll breeze through winter without a cold, just as I did this year; and that you can spark up your metabolism and burn more calories, helping you to get fit with greater ease. You may wake up one day knowing you feel much stronger than you did and have a greater sense of well-being. I want you to say good-bye to poor health, ailments, and chronic diseases because you've chosen the abundant lifestyle.

RAW SOUP TO THE RESCUE! THE SUPERIOR BENEFITS OF A LIVING FOODS DIET

A diet that is made up of a very high percentage of live foods is a healing diet. This is where souping comes in: it helps make eating living foods simple. You simply blend up live ingredients and enjoy.

The living foods diet has helped many people heal their bodies. I see this transformation take place every time my husband and I hold one of our juice and raw-foods retreats. Many people find healing in just one week with us. This diet also transforms your face. Talk about anti-aging! If you want to look younger and have more color in your face, make raw food a large percentage of your diet. Raw foods are rich in anti-aging nutrients such as vitamin C, which supports your collagen, which is that layer just under the skin that is responsible for the youthful look. And look no further when it comes to your DNA. Raw foods give your cells the assistance to transform right down to the DNA level. A healthy cell equals a healthy body.

WHAT LIVING FOODS OFFER YOU

There's an abundance of goodness in living foods. Here's a look at what you get:

Alkalinity

The typical American diet is very acid forming. Foods that turn acidic when metabolized include grains, animal protein, sweets, coffee, alcohol, sodas, and black tea. This creates a slightly acidic internal environment in your body where parasites and yeast can multiply and cancer cells can thrive. When we eat too many acid-forming foods and not enough alkaline-forming foods, our bodies will retain too many acids, storing them in fat cells to protect your delicate tissues and organs. This makes it difficult to lose weight because the body hangs on to the fat cells to protect you. The most alkalizing foods are vegetables and live foods made out of them, including raw soups and veggie juices, as well as sprouts, seeds, and nuts. This makes soup your alkalizing friend.

Hydration

When you overly cook food, it loses a lot of the water. Since your body is made up of a large percentage of water, you need to replenish the water daily. Eating raw foods help to hydrate your body along with providing an abundance of nutrients. The better hydrated you are, the more energized your body.

Abundance of vitamins and minerals

When you cook food, you lose a great deal of vitamins. And when you steam veggies, minerals get leached away. When you make cooked soup, you keep the minerals, however. And when you make raw soup, you retain both the vitamins and minerals.

Biophotons

Raw soups and juices are also loaded with biophotons, which are light rays of energy plants absorb from the sun. When foods are cooked, those light rays are destroyed. The more biophotons a plant absorbs, the more beneficial that plant is for your cells. Biophotons feed the mitochondria—the energy units of your cells that produce ATP, the energy fuel. If you are lacking energy, eat more raw foods, and blend some up in a great souping recipe. These photons help your cells communicate more effectively and help to regulate them.[3]

Enzymes

One of the benefits of live or raw foods is enzymes. They are key to good health because they are part of almost every chemical reaction that takes place in the body. They work with hormones. They pair up with minerals and are partners with vitamins. These lovely little plant enzymes assist the digestive system because they predigest food. This spares the pancreas and other digestive organs a lot of extra work because they don't have to produce as many enzymes for digestion. So the next time you soup it up with a lovely blended drink made with greens, fruits, nuts, or sprouts, just remember you are flooding your body with enzymes, which is very transformative.

Gentle detoxification

The antioxidants and other nutrients in raw foods help the body gently detoxify. You get phytonutrients and antioxidants that bind to free radicals and other toxins and carry them out of the body so they don't damage cells.

A Story of Life

A client came to me a number of years ago in a life-threatening situation. She had gained fifty pounds of water weight and no one knew how to help her. There was no clear diagnosis as to what was wrong with her, but she was so tired and ill she could not even walk down her driveway to the mailbox. It was impossible for her to clean her house. Both her allopathic doctor and her naturopathic doctor had given up. They each told her she should get her affairs in order because she did not have long to live. When I counseled her, I told her as long as she was here, I had hope she could recover. I told her to add a green drink (or a green blended drink) before each meal. Her meals were healthy, so she didn't need to change them. Several months later I heard from her. She was a brand-new person. She lost all that water weight. Her body came into harmony. She was able to walk a mile a day, chop firewood, and clean her house and her garage.

That's what living foods can do! Are you interested?

SOUPER INGREDIENTS

We have looked at the general benefits of living foods. Now let's look at the specific benefits of some of the most often used soup ingredients and how they affect your health. Cater the specific ingredients you use most often for your own specific health issues and needs. This can really make a difference in your health. In addition, remember that if you are making cooked soup, you can add some of the vegetables toward the end of the simmering time to preserve more of the nutrients. But as you'll learn in this section, some of these foods and their specific nutrients are best absorbed when they are cooked.

Arugula

Arugula is replete with antioxidants. It has been found to lower the risk of cancer, help keep bones healthy, improve eyesight, increase metabolic functions, boost the immune system, help with mineral absorption, and strengthen cognitive functions. Also known as rocket salad, this leafy green plant is found throughout the world and belongs in the same family as cauliflower, cabbage, kale, and brussels sprouts. Arugula's high concentration of vitamins (including vitamin A, various B vitamins, vitamin C, and vitamin K) and minerals (including potassium, manganese, iron, and calcium) play a key role in maintaining overall health and preventing various diseases. The high levels of antioxidants found in this plant help in the ongoing fight against free radicals that have been implicated in the aging process, while the high concentration of carotenoids help vision to remain healthy as a person ages. The peppery flavor makes arugula a favorite substitute for lettuce and an exciting addition to soups, salads, and savory dishes.[4]

Asparagus

Asparagus, a nutrient-dense vegetable originating in Africa, Asia, and Europe, is consumed for the delicate flavor in the stocks. This plant is an excellent source for vitamin A, various B vitamins, vitamin C, vitamin E, vitamin K, folate, copper, selenium, fiber, manganese, magnesium, phosphorus, potassium, choline, zinc, iron, pantothenic acid, calcium, selenium, the antioxidant flavonoid rutin, and many different phytonutrient compounds. It is also a good source of protein. The food may be used effectively to prevent or treat a variety of ailments, including cancer, diabetes, cataracts, arthritis, tuberculosis, neurodegenerative diseases, convulsions, urinary tract infections, blood cholesterol, premenstrual syndrome, and menstrual cramps. Research also suggests that asparagus can help as an anti-inflammatory and assist with fertility, healthy pregnancies, digestive health, and cardiovascular health. The wealth of antioxidants in asparagus have the potential to treat oxidative stress.[5]

Basil

Basil is one of the most popular culinary herbs, and with good reason. Its unique and delicious flavor couples well with other foods, in addition to aiding in the digestive process. It eases gas and stomach cramps and can even be taken to relieve nausea and vomiting. This helpful herb is also prized as an anti-inflammatory aid to joints. It has antimicrobial properties and is helpful in preventing diabetes and cardiovascular disease. Basil essential oils may lower blood glucose, triglycerides, and cholesterol. Along with its use as a culinary herb, basil is used as a tea and as a poultice (for mosquito and other insect bites). Basil is a reliable source of manganese, copper, vitamin A, vitamin C, vitamin K, calcium, folate, iron, omega-3 fats, and magnesium.[6]

Beets

Beets are an excellent source of betalains, which help with detoxification. Beets also have antioxidants and help with inflammation. Beets may even help with cancer: "In recent lab studies on human tumor cells, betanin pigments from beets have been shown to lessen tumor cell growth through a number of mechanisms, including inhibition of pro-inflammatory enzymes (specifically, cyclooxygenase enzymes)."[7] Beets have been used to help treat a variety of ailments ever since the Middle Ages. And studies have shown that even just one glass of beet juice per day can reduce blood pressure a significant amount.[8]

Beet greens

Beet greens are a rich source of non-heme iron. They are also one of the best sources of the carotenoids lutein and beta-carotene. They contain a fair amount of protein, phosphorus, and zinc as well as fiber. And they are packed with antioxidants that help your body in detoxification. Studies indicate that beet greens are rich in vitamin K, which is a key nutrient to help prevent osteoporosis. It works with calcium to improve bone health. It also plays a role in fighting Alzheimer's disease.[9]

Broccoli

Broccoli is rich in vitamin C and sulforaphane, and these benefits have better retention when broccoli is lightly steamed. Therefore, if you are making a raw soup, lightly steam broccoli before blending it; if you are making a cooked soup, add the broccoli toward the end of simmering. Because of the sulforaphane, broccoli offers anti-inflammatory benefits. One study showed that participants eating 1.66 cups of steamed broccoli per day for ten days experienced a reduction in C-reactive protein (CRP), one of the markers for heart disease, and lutein and folate. It has also been used to rev up our inflammatory response for short-term healing of injury. It is also rich in a phytonutrient known as kaempferol, which helps improve reactions to allergens. Broccoli also improves detoxification, so it would be good to include in detox soup recipes. It has also been shown to lower the risk of a variety of cancers if you consume ½ cup per day. In addition it's been shown to offer digestive and cardio-vascular support.[10]

Brussels sprouts

Brussels sprouts offer cholesterol-reduction benefits if they are lightly steamed. One study showed that they offer DNA protection when consuming 1¼ cups per day. They also offer glucosinolates, which are phytonutrients that help to protect us from developing cancer. Brussels sprouts support the detoxification system. They offer an array of antioxidants and a sulfur-containing compound D3T that optimizes our detoxification system. They also

offer anti-inflammatory properties and support the digestive system and cardiovascular system.[11]

Cabbage

Cabbage contains about twenty different antioxidant
flavonoids and fifteen different phenols along with many
anti-inflammatory nutrients. Red cabbage specifically
offers anthocyanin antioxidants, beta-carotene, and lutein.
Cabbage also contains sinigrin, a sulfur-containing glucosinolate that has been identified in cancer prevention
research.[12] It has also been found in a study in Denmark
to help prevent type 2 diabetes.[13] It also supports the cardiovascular and digestive systems.

Carrots

Carrots are one of the most used vegetables in the
world because they are so easy to grow and lend themselves to a wide variety of dishes. This root vegetable
is a rich source of antioxidants, vitamins, and minerals,
including vitamins A, C, K, B; pantothenic acid; folate;
potassium; iron; copper; and manganese. Because of their
high levels of beta-carotene, carrots are a popular way of
improving vision, lowering the risk of macular degenera-
tion, and preventing night blindness. Beta-carotene consumption can also reduce the risk of cancer, especially
lung, colon, and breast cancers. Carrots have also been
found to improve cholesterol, reduce hypertension, and
help the immune system. High levels of dietary fiber and
a saliva-producing agent contained in this vegetable aid
digestion, thereby improving oral and gastrointestinal

health. This is also a diabetic-friendly vegetable as it is an effective regulator of blood sugar levels.[14]

Cauliflower

Cauliflower is a popular cruciferous vegetable that is rich in sulfur-containing compounds. Found in the Mediterranean region, it is high in glucosinolates and flavonoids, phytonutrients that support our cardiovascular health, digestive tract, immune system, inflammatory system, and detoxification systems. Studies have shown that cooking cauliflower improves its ability to bind with bile acids. Cauliflower contains the antioxidants beta-carotene, beta-cryptoxanthin, caffeic acid, cinnamic acid, ferulic acid, quercetin, rutin, and kaempferol. Cauliflower is considered a cancer-preventative vegetable that is high in fiber and excellent for the digestive tract.[15]

Celery

Evidence shows that celery was used as a medicinal plant in ancient Egypt. Today, though, it's thought of as a crunchy veggie stick on a vegetable plate with dip or a part of soup and without a big nutritional punch. But this is far from the truth. Current research has shown its anti-inflammatory effects and especially inflammation in the digestive system. Scientists have identified many antioxidants in celery that help reduce damage done to the body's fat and blood vessels. Celery has often been singled out for its high sodium content, and people on a low-sodium diet were told to avoid it.[16] But the sodium in celery and table salt (sodium chloride) are not anything alike. Most people are deficient in organic sodium. Sodium is sometimes called the "youth mineral" because it promotes healthy joints. Sodium is also very alkaline, which helps neutralize the acids produced from a stressful lifestyle and by eating too many acid-forming foods.[17]

Chard

Both ancient Greeks and ancient Romans used chard for its medicinal properties. Its phytonutrients offer special benefits for blood sugar control. Chard is a good source of betalains, which are phytonutrients that offer antioxidants, act as an anti-inflammatory, and help with detoxification. It's actually one of the most nutritious vegetables. It's very rich in vitamin K and magnesium, which are excellent support for the bones. Vitamin K_2 activates osteocalcin, the protein in bones that helps keep calcium in the bones.[18]

Cilantro

Cilantro is an herb that originated in the Mediterranean and Asia Minor. It adds great flavor to many dishes from salsa to curry. Cilantro is rich in a variety of phytonutrients along with vitamins A, C, and K.[19] It has been found to suppress lead accumulation in animal studies and is known for its ability to chelate, thus detoxify, lead as well as other metals from the body.[20] It's helpful to reduce anxiety. It helps the urinary tract fight off infections.[21] With all these wonderful benefits, why not toss some cilantro into most of your soup recipes?

Corn

If you thought corn was just a starchy vegetable, you're in for a nice surprise. I'm from Iowa, and I grew up on sweet corn. It tastes so great that I wondered how it could be very healthful. What a nice surprise to learn that it has nutritional value. Yellow corn is rich in the carotenoids lutein and zeaxanthin along with a variety of other phytonutrients. Corn is also a good source of fiber. And a lectin in corn has been shown to have HIV-inhibiting properties.[22]

Cucumber

Cucumbers have been used throughout history for their hydrating and cooling effects. Just as the desert dwellers knew, cucumbers are refreshing on a hot summer day. Try a refreshing cold cucumber soup. I also love cucumbers for juicing because they provide a lot of juice. They are a natural diuretic. They have antioxidant and anti-inflammatory properties. And they also have special phytonutrients that have been studied for their anticancer properties.[23]

Garlic

Garlic was prescribed by Hippocrates, sometimes known as father of medicine, for a variety of diseases and illnesses. Garlic was even used as a performance enhancer for athletes in Ancient Greece. "According to the National Library of Medicine, part of the NIH (National Institutes of Health), USA, garlic is widely used for several conditions linked to the blood system and heart, including atherosclerosis (hardening of the arteries), high cholesterol, heart attack, coronary heart disease and hypertension."[24] Garlic has been a long-used remedy for colds and flu because of its natural antibiotic properties. Be sure to include it in soup especially when you feel a bug trying to get you down.

Ginger

Beyond its use in cooking and popular beverages the world over, ginger is also widely regarded as a potent medicinal herb. Ginger has treated humanity therapeutically for thousands of years. A powerhouse of healthy energy, it is known to improve circulation in the body and lower blood-level triglycerides connected with diabetes and cardiovascular disease. Because of ginger's ability to protect the immune system, it is a popular remedy for colds, congestion, influenza, and sore throat. It is frequently used to treat food poisoning, nausea, indigestion, motion sickness, and vomiting. It has been shown to be effective against acids and toxins in the gastrointestinal tract.[25]

Green beans

Green beans are one of the main sources of nutrients for peoples throughout the world. Known by a variety of names, including french beans and string beans, this vegetable helps reduce the risk of heart disease and colon cancer, regulate digestive processes, eliminate harmful free radicals from the body, and keep the eyes and bones healthy. These benefits are the result of green beans being full of immune system–boosting antioxidants, fiber, vitamins (A, B$_6$, C, K, and folic acid) and minerals (calcium, silicon, iron, manganese, potassium, and copper). Green beans come in around 150 different varieties and can be grown in most climates of the world.[26]

Kale

Kale is a cruciferous vegetable that has been studied for its cancer prevention benefits. It also offers antioxidant and anti-inflammatory benefits. It also helps to lower cholesterol. Kale's isothiocyanates support the body's detoxification system. It also supports our digestive system. It's very high in vitamin K, which is important for bone strength.[27]

Legumes

Legumes are a family of plants featuring a pod with seeds inside it. Also referred to as pulses, it includes peas, beans, peanuts, and lentils. Legumes are one of the best sources of protein on the planet, in addition to being rich in fiber. They also contain an array of various vitamins and minerals, including iron, zinc, magnesium, vitamin A, vitamin K, and various B vitamins. Legumes help to keep cholesterol levels low, stabilize digestion, promote cardiac health, regulate glucose levels in the blood, help prevent or remedy constipation, and aid in weight management.[28] The most important members of the legume family are lentils, which have an impressive array of health benefits in addition to offering energy without significant increase in calories.[29]

Nettles

Although nettle is often thought of as simply an annoying weed, the ancient Greeks and Romans actually cultivated nettle for both food and medicine. From ancient to modern times, nettle has been used in a myriad of healing applications including anemia, dermatological problems, gout, rheumatism, exhaustion, joint discomfort, menstrual ailments, fertility issues, menopausal symptoms, prostate health, and liver health. Nettle can be cooked and eaten as a nourishing food or made into a tea. Nettles contain vitamin C, vitamin E, beta-carotene (vitamin A), along with vitamins B_1, B_2, B_3, and B_5. Nettles are also rich in minerals, including calcium, potassium, magnesium, phosphorus, and iron. They are also a valued source of protein, fat, and fiber. This plant is famously known for its ability to produce a sting when handled due to the presence of formic acid in its sharp, fine protrusions. However, the formic acid is easily destroyed after harvesting by either heating or drying the leaves.[30]

Onion

Onions make just about any cooked soup taste better. But they also offer a package of nutrition. Here's a little tip when chopping them up for your soup: peel off as little of the onion as possible because the flavonoids are concentrated in the outer layers. "A red onion can lose about 20% of its quercetin and almost 75% of its antocyanins" if too much is removed. Onions help regulate blood fats and cholesterol. Eating onions several times a week can lower your risk of cancer. One of the most prevalent nutrients in onions is biotin, which is great for hair growth.[31]

Oregano

Oregano is so much more than a classic and flavorful culinary herb. It is an incredibly powerful healing plant with antibacterial properties that has been used historically to treat a wide variety of bodily ailments. Oregano contains two volatile oils: thymol and carvacrol. These oils, present in the whole food integrity of wild oregano, inhibit the growth of bacteria such as Staphylococcus aureus and Pseudomonas aeruginosa. They are also known to keep the fungus Candida albicans in check. Oregano has been known to relieve or prevent colds, influenza, headaches, menstrual cramping, and respiratory illness. Oregano has been prized for its ability to protect against free-radical damage in the human body. Oregano is a source of vitamin B_6, vitamin E, folate, calcium, iron, and magnesium.[32]

Parsley

This nutritious Mediterranean plant was prized by the ancient Greeks. It was originally used exclusively as a medicinal plant and only later for food. Some of the ancient uses of this plant include being used to treat toothaches, bruises, insect bites, and rough skin. Because of parsley's anti-inflammatory properties it can work as a pain reliever, in addition to strengthening the immune system, offering relief from indigestion, stomach cramps, bloating, and nausea. As modern scientists have begun studying this amazing plant, they have found it full of vitamins A, B, C, E, K, beta-carotene, pantothenic acid, choline, folates, calcium, iron, magnesium, manganese, phosphorous, potassium, zinc, copper, as well as various constituents that have anticarcinogenic, anti-inflammatory, antidiabetic, and antiarthritis properties.[33]

Peas

Although the green pea is often overlooked, it is actually one of the healthiest foods in the world. Scientists are still learning about the health benefits of this vegetable, which was one of the very first foods to be cultivated and can survive in nearly every climate. Green peas contain some phytonutrients not found in other foods, as well as nutrients high in antioxidant and anti-inflammatory benefits. Green peas are also an excellent source of fiber; calcium; iron; copper; zinc; manganese; vitamins B, C, E, and K; folate; and alpha-linolenic acid (ALA). Interestingly many commercial protein powders are starting to use green peas because they contain such a high concentration of quality protein.[34]

Rosemary

Although this perennial herb is most frequently associated with its delicious taste and fragrant aroma, it actually has a vast array of health benefits that have been largely forgotten in the modern world. Native to Mediterranean regions, rosemary has the ability to improve mood, boost memory, increase intelligence, and relieve pain. Modern science has discovered that rosemary is full of antioxidant as well as anti-inflammatory, antibacterial, and anticarcinogenic properties. When rosemary leaves or essential oil are added to food or applied topically, it can help reduce inflammation, boost the immune system and circulation, help with detoxification, promote healthy skin, act as an antiaging treatment, and protect the body from bacterial infections and other illnesses and diseases.[35]

Spinach

Spinach is rich in chlorophyll, a blood purifier. It is a top source of magnesium and iron. It has anti-inflammatory compounds and is a good source of the carotenoids lutein and zeaxanthin. It is also a good source of vitamins A, B_2, B_6, E, and K, and folate. "Several recent studies in this area have shown thylakoid-rich extracts from spinach to delay stomach emptying, decrease levels of hunger-related hormones like ghrelin, and increase levels of satiety-related hormones like glucagon-like peptide 1 (GLP-1)."[36]

Thyme

Thyme is an evergreen shrub originating in parts of Africa and the Mediterranean. It has been prized for thousands of years for its medicinal properties. There is a reference to thyme in one of the oldest known medical books, the Egyptian *Ebers Papyrus*, dating from sixteenth century BC. The Ancient Greeks also prized this herb and used it in their temples because of its rich aromatic quality. It isn't surprising that thyme has been so highly esteemed throughout history, considering that it has one of the highest antioxidant concentrations of any herb. These antioxidant properties help prevent the oxidative stress that causes the various systems of the body to wear down over time. Thyme is also a powerhouse of iron, potassium, manganese, and a variety of other essential minerals. Thyme contains thymol, an organic compound used in mouthwashes and various personal hygiene products because of its antifungal and antiseptic properties. In cooking it is hard to go wrong with thyme, as its subtle and comforting flavor can be used to enhance the flavor of almost any dish. Thyme can be used whole or with the leaves removed from the stems, and it can also be ground into a spice or used as an essential oil.[37]

Tomato

Tomato has been most widely studied for its lycopene, which can unequivocally lower prostate cancer risk in men. And lycopene is more bioavailable when cooked. It's also been studied regarding small-cell lung cancer, pancreatic cancer, and breast cancer. Tomatoes also play a part in bone health. Also, phytonutrients found in tomatoes were shown to help prevent clumping of platelet cells. Tomatoes are an excellent source of vitamin C along with beta-carotene, lutein, and zeaxanthin.[38]

Watercress

Watercress is a powerful food that is believed to have been carried by Roman soldiers on their journeys because of its health properties.[39] Studies show it's been linked to lowering high cholesterol levels. A 2008 study gave rats watercress for thirty days. The results were promising: "Rats were able to normalize their triglycerides, cholesterol levels, and LDL, while raising their HDL," which is good cholesterol.[40] Like beet juice, "watercress contains a high level of dietary nitrate."[41] Studies have shown these nitrates can reduce blood pressure. In a study those who ate watercress lowered their "diastolic blood pressure by an average of 3.7 mm Hg in just three days."[42] Watercress is also "rich in a specific glucosinolate known as gluconasturtiin," which helps prevent cancer by keeping blood vessels from forming for tumors.[43] Last but not least, watercress also helps manage diabetes. Regularly eating watercress may help blood sugar balance for diabetes and prediabetes.[44]

Zucchini

Initially zucchini is rich in antioxidants and a particularly good source of vitamin C. It is also a good source of potassium, which helps to lower blood pressure. Zucchini has been recommended for digestive issues and leaky gut syndrome because of its anti-inflammatory protection.[45] A study published in 2008 found polyphenols and ascorbic acid in the peels that benefited thyroid, adrenal, and insulin regulation.[46]

WHAT LIVING FOODS HAVE GIVEN ME

I'm quite sure that living foods saved my life. Raw foods, including blended raw soups and juices, have given my body energy and healing nutrients through all my challenges. Many days after the attack I was so tired that I felt like I could barely move. But by pouring in live foods day after day, I felt energy returning. Now when I feel tired or get that afternoon lull, a raw soup or juice is a great pick-me-up. I encourage you to give it try. It really does work.

A LIVE-FOOD SOUP RECIPE

CHERIE'S AWESOME GREEN SOUP

1 cup carrot juice (5–7 large carrots)
1 avocado, peeled
1 handful spinach
¼–½ tsp. cumin

Put all the ingredients in a blender and process until smooth. Enjoy! Serves 1.

LIVE FOOD WILL GIVE YOU LIFE!

When you include more living foods in your diet, such as what you find in raw soups and blended drinks, you help your metabolism to hum along efficiently. You'll also help your body detoxify, which you'll learn more about in the next chapter. People who do not eat enough live food are far more likely to suffer from fatigue, weight gain, poor skin, food allergies, heartburn, intestinal problems, sleep issues, and constipation. Your colon needs high-fiber live food to move the waste along. And you need enzymes from live food to facilitate your digestion. Not eating enough live food can lead to malnutrition, which promotes illness and a compromised immune system. Therefore incorporating more raw soups into your diet can greatly help in your desire to get more live foods into your diet. I want you to experience all the great benefits and rewards of feeling really alive, happy, and engaged with life. Live foods can make a big difference for you. Happy souping!

CHAPTER 4

DETOXING WITH SOUP

"Yes," said Cook. "That is soup that you are smelling. The princess, not that you would know or care, is missing, bless her goodhearted self. And times are terrible. And when times are terrible, soup is the answer. Don't it smell like the answer?"[1]

—KATE DICAMILLO

SOUP CAN BE an integral part of any detox program. Warm soup is especially good when the weather is cool. Raw blended soup is ideal anytime. If you are doing a liquid fast, consider adding blended vegan soups to your menu. There are many detox combinations that will facilitate your cleansing program.

With souping for detox in mind, think about your body for a minute as you would your car. What if you never changed the oil or filters in your car? You know what would happen. When I got my first car, which was a cute little yellow VW bug, I somehow missed the lesson from my dad about changing the oil every three thousand miles. I just drove and drove that cute little car until it died on a Southern California freeway in rush-hour traffic. That was a harrowing experience!

Our bodies are a bit like our cars. They have filter systems that need to be cleaned out and fluids that need to be flushed out. That's where souping comes in with fresh, live blended and juiced drinks, along with gently warmed soups, and yes, even the simmered-all-day soups can help you detoxify your body. You see, they all offer an abundance of antioxidants, which bind to toxins and help your body carry them out.

We're bombarded by pollution along with a host of toxic stuff in our food such as preservatives, dyes, fillers, and additives. Experts estimate that between 5 pounds and 10 pounds of accumulated toxic waste is in our cells, tissues, and organs, particularly in our colon. Toxins in the brain can cause a host of cognitive and emotional problems, such as brain fog, depression, and emotional outbursts. They make us weak, restless, and unable to fight off infections. They can even cause pain in our muscles and joints. Have you ever eaten something that was artificially sweetened and flavored, meaning it was loaded with toxic substances, and noticed a day or two later that your back or muscles ached or your feet were sore? Toxic molecules, known as free radicals, damage our cells, creating numerous health problems along with aches and pains. And they accelerate aging. All this stuff creates internal toxic soup. This is why it's so crucial to periodically cleanse your body.

On a detox program we can get rid of toxic substances, excess mucus, and waste. A lot of this toxic stuff gets stored in fat cells because that's the safest place to put it, but the bad news is that this can keep us from losing weight. The body hangs on to the fat to protect our delicate tissues and organs. But when nutrient-rich soups come along in abundance, as it will with a soup detox program, the body says, "OK, I can let go of this stuff now because the antioxidant infantry is here to escort the bad things out."

Not only will detoxing help you lose weight, but it will also help you heal your body and get well, if that's your goal. Toxins make us sick and keep us from getting well. If you aren't feeling well, it's time for a major detox. This chapter will show you how to incorporate soup into a detox program. (For the complete detox programs for each of the organs of elimination, see my book *Juicing, Fasting, and Detoxing for Life* or join my online program 30-Day Detox.)

When your pathways of elimination get choked with toxins and they can't do their work efficiently, you need to detox. Here's how the scenario goes. The colon gets clogged with mucus and waste that doesn't get eliminated. This can turn to a hardened, rubberlike substance that keeps the nutrients from being properly absorbed. Instead, toxins get absorbed back into the system. The liver gets overwhelmed with all the toxic substances it has to filter. It can become congested and even develop stones or become fatty. Likewise the kidneys can fall behind in filtering out toxins, some of which can get recirculated. Also, the skin, which is our largest organ of elimination, can show symptoms of toxic buildup with rashes, pimples, acne, eczema, or other conditions. Then toxins collect in cells, organs, and bodily fluids between the cells. Cellular metabolism becomes inefficient. That's when lumps of trapped toxins, water, and fat show up as the lumpy tissue we call cellulite.

THE CELLULITE SOUP CURE

What causes that lumpy, bumpy orange-peel-looking stuff called cellulite? Well for starters, it's not just another lump of pudge. Cellulite is a mix of lymph, fluids, toxins, and waste. No one thinks these dimples are cute, and most of us know that exercise doesn't erase the dimples off our hips, thighs, or buttocks. And the most oft-asked question is, "How do I get rid of it?"

To get rid of cellulite, you must tackle it in a completely different way than regular fat. It starts with detoxing to remove the toxins. You also must address constipation and improve lymphatic drainage. It is important to strengthen weak blood vessels throughout this process. In doing all this, you will make it easier for your body to burn the fat in those areas. Constipation causes toxins to remain in the system and circulate throughout the body; they then affect organs such as the kidneys and liver. The lymphatic system doesn't have a pump, so moving the

lymph, which is the waste-carrying channel, is impera-
tive. Exercise, massage, and lymphatic cleansing are the
only ways to cleanse the lymphatic system along with
a lymphasizer, which is a machine designed to move
lymph. (See the appendix.)

A poor diet that includes refined flour products, sugar,
junk food, refined salt (sodium chloride), coffee, black
tea, alcohol, tobacco, bad fats, and oils all contribute to
a congested lymphatic system and liver. It also impacts
the circulatory system. Then it becomes more difficult for
your body to get rid of cellulite, and it can even cause it
to form. It is believed that toxins are the top reason cellulite forms in the first place.

The frustrating part for many people is that you can't
get rid of cellulite just by eating a healthy diet and exercising. You can't rub it off with creams and lotions or melt
if off with seaweed wraps. It will only disappear as you
internally cleanse your liver, colon, and lymphatic system.
You must also improve your circulation and metabolism
and get your lymphatic system moving. It also helps to
nourish your body with living foods through raw soups
and juices. This will give you the best chance to get rid
of lumps and bulges.

Can cleansing with soup help? Absolutely! A total
body cleanse is your path to fewer dimples and smoother
skin. Making your first step to get rid of toxins be a soup
detox plan can be very beneficial. I know firsthand that
this works. Plain and simple, if you want to be cellulite-
free, you have to flush out the toxins. It's also important

to nourish and condition your body with a variety of nutrients in your soups. This will help you strengthen blood vessels, an important step in ridding your body of cellulite. Cleansing away toxins will also help improve your circulation. As you remove the toxins and trapped water, strengthen blood vessels so that fluids don't leak into surrounding spaces, and nourish your tissues with an abundance of nutrients, you will see cellulite melt away.

During one of my 30-Day Detox programs, one young woman e-mailed to say, "Wow!" She had looked in the mirror one day and all her cellulite was gone. She couldn't believe it because she hadn't even been exercising—just doing the cleanse. And she ended up cellulite-free.

If you want more information on how to get rid of cellulite, get my e-book titled *The Cellulite Cure*, which is available on my website. It could help you experience freedom from the dimples.

ARE YOU TOXIC?

Have you ever wondered about how many toxins might be hiding out in your body? Take the toxicity quiz below. If you need to detox, you can start with the soup detox plans found later in this chapter.

Toxicity quiz

Check off the symptoms that describe you. If you note even a few points, I suggest you detox.

☐ Aches and pains

☐ Acid reflux

☐ Arthritis

☐ Bloating and gas

☐ Cellulite

☐ Constipation

☐ Dizziness

☐ Emotional and mental problems

☐ Headaches

☐ Hormone imbalances

☐ Inability to lose weight

☐ Indigestion

☐ Irritability

☐ Lack of energy and fatigue

☐ Excess weight

☐ Premature aging

☐ Restlessness

☐ Sinus problems

☐ Skin problems

☐ Stressful feelings

☐ Trouble sleeping/insomnia

☐ Visual problems

☐ Weakness

THE SOUPER DETOX PROGRAMS

Rather than show you just a general overall cleanse, which is fine by the way, I will show you how to cleanse and support the various organs of elimination with the fabulous nutrients in the soups. This program can be used alone for a gentle cleanse or can be combined with herbal cleanse products and various other supplements to get a more thorough cleansing. This will revive your organs, blood, and systems of elimination.

As I mentioned in chapter 1, my first cleanse was a five-day juice fast. On the fifth day my body expelled a tumor the size of a golf ball. That's a notable benefit for a cleanse, wouldn't you say! You can get good results with raw blended soups, which I also call smoothies. I've used smoothies, raw soups, and juices for many cleanses that I have done through the years. Soups give you a bit more substance, which helps your stamina when you're working. And in the late fall and winter months, hot soups will help to warm your body inside out. I've also done cleanses when I had a soup for every meal. That feels very nurturing.

I'll never forget one cleanse when I had a pitcher of beet

juice sitting in the refrigerator for several small glasses of beet juice for my husband and me to drink during the day. He forgot what the program was and drank the whole pitcher. Beet juice is quite cleansing, so I saw very little of him for several hours. That's a humorous moment, but most of my cleanses haven't been that eventful. But what is noteworthy is how I feel afterward—alive, refreshed, rejuvenated, and restored to vibrant health.

GET STARTED WITH THE COLON-CLEANSE PROGRAM

I recommend you do a colon cleanse before you do any other organ or system detox. It's very important that you have a cleared intestinal tract before detoxing other systems so that when other organs begin dumping toxins, they can be eliminated easily.

So first, let's look at why colon cleansing is so important. Then we'll look at how soups, and particularly raw soups, can help you cleanse your colon.

Why do a colon cleanse?

When you eat junk food, processed fare, a lot of cooked food, fried foods, sweets, coffee, sweetened lattes, sports drinks, soda pop (no pop is good, but diet is the worst), alcohol, candy, cake, cookies, ice cream, or drugs (prescription and recreational), mucous secretions get stimulated and coat your intestinal lining. This is an innate process designed to protect the delicate tissues of the intestinal tract from irritating substances, such as toxic waste or spoiled food. This protective mechanism was only meant for an occasional episode, not a continual onslaught. When we constantly eat substances that are irritating to our elimination tract, mucus and waste material will build up and coat the lining. It can turn into a hard, rubbery plaque called mucoid plaque. This can become a nice breeding ground where parasites and yeast can hide and thrive. And the absorption of nutrients is impaired as the majority of our nutrients are absorbed through the intestines.

Symptoms of a toxic colon

Below is a list of the symptoms you may experience if you have a toxic colon. Check off any symptoms you experience:[2]

- ☐ Bloating

- ☐ Constipation

- ☐ Diarrhea

- ☐ Difficulty digesting foods

- ☐ Diseases and disorders including irritable bowel syndrome (IBS), acid reflux and heartburn (GERD), Crohn's disease, diverticulitis, Candida albicans, leaky gut syndrome, food allergies, lactose intolerance, hemorrhoids, polyps, and colon cancer

- ☐ Exhaustion

☐ Foul-smelling stools or gas

☐ Frequent colds and/or headaches

☐ Gas

☐ Gluten sensitivity

☐ Irritability

☐ Mood swings

☐ Parasites

☐ Rashes or skin conditions

☐ Stomach pain

☐ Weight gain and difficulty losing weight

If you experience even just one or a few of these, it may be time to do a colon cleanse.

Souper colon cleansing

Souper cleansing to the rescue! It's time to get out your blender and soup pot. Include more of these foods in your soups, especially the raw soups:

- Greens. Raw green veggies offer your body the enzymes and minerals, such as magnesium, that help cleanse your colon of insufficiently digested food and mucoid plaque. As we age, the body produces less stomach acid and digestive enzymes, which leads to less efficient digestion. Cooking destroys enzymes, so make sure most of your soups are raw, and add greens such as chard, kale, spinach, parsley, and collard greens. You can blend up lots of veggies such as cucumber and zucchini for raw soups.

- Foods high in chlorophyll. Chlorophyll, which is what gives vegetables their green color, promotes colon cleansing because it is a fat-soluble nutrient that clings to the lining of the intestinal wall and curbs bacterial growth while also helping to remove harmful bacteria. It also helps to heal the mucosal linking of the intestinal tract. Vegetables high in chlorophyll include asparagus, brussels sprouts, cabbage, celery, collard greens, chard, leeks, peas, and spinach. Each of these would make a good addition to your soup.

- Garlic. This spice has antiviral, antiparasitic, and antibacterial properties, meaning that it helps remove pathogens from the intestinal tract. It also has anti-inflammatory properties, and it helps in removing toxins and waste.

- Lemon is very cleansing for your entire system. It can have antiseptic effects on

the intestinal tract along with halting the
growth of microorganisms.

- Avocado has beneficial oils that assist
  with digestion.

Vegetables are, as you can tell, one of the most important aspects of a colon cleanse. Make sure your soups
have some of the vegetables listed below in them; they
are the best vegetables for a colon cleanse:

- Asparagus

- Brussels sprouts

- Cabbage

- Carrots

- Celery

- Collard greens

- Dark leafy greens such as spinach, kale,
  watercress, and arugula

- Sea vegetables

- Swiss chard

When I did my first colon cleanse with raw blended
soups and juices, I also included fiber shakes and herbal
remedies that helped me get rid of a lot of old waste and
toxic material. When I was finished, I looked about ten

years younger and much more vibrant. I've had a number of people report weight loss and getting rid of belly fat and bloating after completing a colon cleanse.

Menu plan

Juice and soup fast

Drink 3–5 glasses (or bowls/cups) of raw soups, smoothies, and juice each day for three to seven days. Choose recipes from chapter 8, and be sure to use some of the vegetables already mentioned. You may choose to go on a one- to five-day soup and vegetable juice fast. This will greatly facilitate the colon-cleanse process. Soups should be raw and blended as much as possible. In cold weather you can add a cup or two of warm soup to the program to keep you warm.

Hydration

Drink at least eight glasses of purified water each day.

Hot water, lemon, and cayenne

It is nice to start your day with a hot drink. During a colon cleanse, it is helpful to begin your day with the juice of one quarter of a lemon and a sprinkle of cayenne pepper added to hot water. This morning drink will help to stimulate your digestive juices, wake up your liver, and get it moving in the morning. This drink acts a bit like a laxative.

Full colon cleansing option

For the full colon cleansing option, include the following in your plan as well:

- Bentonite clay and fiber: Twice a day—
  morning and evening—mix 1 tablespoon
  of fiber and 1 tablespoon of bentonite
  clay (powder or liquid for internal use)
  in 8 ounces of water. You can put all
  this in a jar or a shaker and shake until
  well combined. Drink as soon as possible
  because it will gel and become very thick.
  Bentonite clay is an edible clay that acts
  as a binding agent that pulls toxic material off the intestinal wall. It will expand
  in the intestinal tract and can collect
  all sorts of toxic material such as pesticides and environmental chemicals, parasites, and old waste and carry them out
  of the colon. The fiber acts like a broom
  sweeping out the waste from the colon.
  Don't be surprised if you see material that
  looks rather old. One caution: this fiber
  shake should be taken two hours apart
  from your medication, or it could interfere
  with absorption of your medication.

- Herbal cleanse: With dinner, take an
  herbal-cleansing product that contains
  such ingredients as Chinese rhubarb
  root, barberry root, dandelion root, fringe
  tree root bark, aronia fruit, chebulic and
  belleric myrobalan fruit, meadowsweet
  aerial plant, English plantain, ginger root,

fennel seed, peppermint leaf, fenugreek seed, and licorice root.

- Probiotics: Take probiotics to replenish the good bacteria in the colon.

- Colon flush: You may wish to do an enema or get a colonic to assist in eliminating wastes.

For intestinal cleanse products that have all the ingredients in the best formulation, see the appendix.

Benefits of colon detoxification

One of the initial benefits you should notice after you've cleansed your colon is that you will have better digestion. When your intestinal tract is overburdened with waste, congestion, and toxins, a lot of energy is used to deal with that just to keep you going. Once the toxins are removed, your body doesn't need to work as hard, and you will also have more energy.

Here are some other benefits you can expect:

- Better health

- Better sleep

- Digestive system cleared of mucus and congestion

- Fewer mood swings

- Greater sense of well-being

- Improved digestion

- Improved skin and younger appearance

- Increased mental clarity

- Lessening or disappearance of pain

- More creativity

- Purified blood

- Recolonization of healthy bacteria

- Reduced cravings for sugar, salt, junk foods, alcohol, and nicotine

- Renewed joy

- Renewed vitality

- Stronger immune system

- Weight loss

Colon-cleansing recipe

COLON CLEANSE GREEN SOUP

½ cup spinach, chopped
¼ cup celery, chopped
½ cup cabbage, chopped
2–3 Tbsp. lime juice (1 lime)
½ avocado
1 cup ice cubes

½ cup senna tea, steeped (optional)
Add water as needed

Blend the ingredients until smooth, add water as needed.
Serve right away. Serves 1.

Note: Senna tea has a laxative effect.

REFRESH YOUR SYSTEM WITH A SOUPER KIDNEY CLEANSE

Your little kidneys perform a mighty job, which includes the following:

- Balancing electrolytes and fluid

- Balancing pH

- Eliminating waste

- Excreting urine

- Regulating blood pressure

What causes kidney congestion and toxicity? It's the typical American diet of sweets and other refined carbohydrates such as bread, rolls, baked goods, sodas, alcohol, overconsumption of animal protein, consumption of damaged fats, and consumption of too many mucus-producing foods such as dairy. Kidney congestion is also caused by eating refined salt (with all minerals except sodium chloride removed), taking drugs, eating foods sprayed with pesticides, eating GMO foods, drinking water with chloride and fluoride, ingesting heavy metals (mercury, aluminum, and lead), radiation, and toxic chemicals in the environment. All these things negatively impact the kidneys and reduce their efficiency. They can lead to more serious problems such as kidney stones or even kidney failure.

One word of caution: if you have a kidney disease, always consult with your doctor before doing a kidney-cleanse program. And if you have an infection, it is wise to see your doctor.

Symptoms of kidney congestion or toxicity

Take a look at the symptoms of kidney congestion and check off any you have:[3]

☐ Seeing bloody and/or cloudy urine

☐ Experiencing burning or pain during urination

☐ Experiencing a cold sensation in the lower half of the body

☐ Having dark circles under the eyes

☐ Urinating frequently, especially at night

☐ Having foul-smelling and/or dark urine

☐ Dealing with incontinence

☐ Feeling pain in or around the eyes

If you have any of these symptoms, you should cleanse your kidneys as soon as possible. To prevent problems with your kidneys, it is an excellent idea to do a kidney cleanse at least once a year.

Helpful ingredients for a kidney cleanse

Using these ingredients in your raw soups and smoothies will help with your kidney cleanse:

- Parsley. This is a good diuretic and often used in kidney cleansing. Mix it with mild-tasting vegetables such as celery, carrot, and cucumber. It is also good with lemon. Make it into a raw soup with more substance by adding an avocado.

- Lemon or lime juice. The citric acid in lemon or lime juice may be helpful in reducing calcium levels in the urine. This can reduce the potential for developing calcium kidney stones.

- Cucumber. This vegetable is an excellent diuretic, and it can be used to make an excellent refreshing cucumber soup.

- Celery. This vegetable increases urine production, which dilutes the toxins and waste in the urine.

- Nettles. Nettles are a natural diuretic that helps to remove impurities, including

bacteria, calcium deposits, and kidney
stones.

- Beets. This vegetable contains betalains,
  which help remove calcium buildup in the
  kidneys.

- Carrots. Carrots help flush out excess uric
  acid, which contributes to kidney stones.

- Radishes. Radishes help the kidneys flush
  out toxins, and radish juice can even help
  dissolve kidney stones.

- Purple cabbage. This vegetable is rich in
  sulfur and vitamin C, which help flush
  out uric acid and free radicals.

Kidney-cleanse menu plan

You should have at least three raw soups and/or juices
each day for three to seven days. Try to use as many of
the ingredients listed above in these soups as you can.
You can have more, but you should not have less.

Here are additions to your soup menu plan that can
help cleanse your kidneys:

- Combine 2 tablespoons of freshly
  squeezed lemon or lime juice and a dash
  of cayenne pepper in 8–10 ounces of purified hot water. Drink this mixture three
  times a day for three days.

- Drink about a gallon of liquid per day. You can make lemon-ginger water by adding the juice of one lemon and about 1 tablespoon of fresh ginger juice to a quart of purified water. You may also drink vegetable juices, purified water, and herbal teas.

- Drink cranberry juice. Studies show that cranberry prevents bacteria from adhering to urinary tract walls. Cranberry juice is also very beneficial for cleansing the kidneys. Drink several glasses of unsweetened cranberry juice mixed with water each day. If you can't find fresh cranberries to juice, get premade unsweetened cranberry juice concentrate or unsweetened cranberry juice and add to water according to taste. You may also add fresh lemon juice and a few drops of stevia or a little apple juice to sweeten, if needed.

- Watermelon juice is also helpful in cleansing the kidneys. Or you can blend watermelon to make watermelon soup. You may also use the rind.

Benefits of cleansing the kidneys

When you cleanse your kidneys and give them nutritional support, they can serve you well. During a kidney cleanse you should get rid of toxins and congestion in these important organs of elimination. When your kidneys have been cleansed and renewed, they will be more efficient at removing toxins from your blood. Here are some specific benefits of a kidney cleanse:

- Balanced blood pressure

- Regulated acids

- Reduced water retention

- Balanced red blood cells (RBCs) by helping the kidneys produce erythropoietin that stimulates the production of RBCs

- Improved waste excretion

- Improved stone-inhibiting substances

- Removal of harmful bacteria and thus prevention of infections

- Release of calcitriol, a hormone that assists the absorption of calcium

- Prevention of kidney failure or kidney disease

Kidney-cleansing recipes

BERRY-BEET KIDNEY DETOX SOUP

1 cup berries (I recommend blueberries or raspberries)
1 organic beet, scrubbed
½ cup unsweetened cranberry juice
½ cup organic almond or coconut milk
2 tsp. organic apple cider vinegar
1 cup dark green leafy vegetables (I recommend chard or kale)
½-inch-chunk ginger root

Blend all ingredients and enjoy! Serves 1.

RADISH AND PURPLE CABBAGE KIDNEY DETOX SOUP

1 cup chopped radish
1 cup chopped purple cabbage
3 ribs capped celery
2–3 Tbsp. lime or lemon juice (approximately 1 lemon or lime)

Blend all ingredients and eat as soon as possible. Serves 1.

THE SOUPER LIVER CLEANSE

A number of years ago a lady with liver problems contacted me; no one had been able to help her. I suggested a liver cleanse starting with raw soups geared toward liver cleansing and freshly made veggies juices made with liver-friendly veggies. In about three weeks she was well. Liver cleansing is one of the best kept secrets of healing. But it shouldn't be a secret. The whole world should know about the restorative benefits of cleansing the liver.

Did you know that the body stores toxins in the liver that can't be eliminated well on a standard diet? There are many toxins in our environment that we get from the air, water, and our food. All the toxins that enter our bodies have to pass through the liver, including pesticides, heavy metals, and harsh chemicals from manufacturing plants. Along with all the chemicals that can impact the liver, so can other substances, such as parasites, yeast/fungus, medications, alcohol, food additives, too much sugar, and viruses. Some toxins are more challenging to get rid of, such as fat-soluble chemicals, which usually get stored in fat cells. For some people even a small amount of toxins can weaken or damage their liver because they are more susceptible and do not have efficient detoxification systems.

There are certain medications that, even taken at the recommended doses, can harm liver cells, namely acetaminophen (Tylenol). Another substance that can cause damage is fructose, which can actually scar the liver. Read labels and especially watch out for high-fructose corn syrup. Agave syrup is not the healthy sweetener people once believed, either; in fact, it is mostly fructose.

No doubt you've heard that alcohol can cause fatty liver and scars in the liver, which can lead to liver cancer.

But did you know that sweets and refined carbs can do the same thing? Fatty liver is on the rise in this country, and many health professionals in the holistic field point to sugar in its many forms and refined carbs as the cause. Also the standard American diet can lead to liver congestion and even stones in the liver.

What about high cholesterol? Have you ever considered that the liver might be involved? The liver makes cholesterol. In fact, it makes more of this substance than you would normally eat. If your cholesterol is on the rise, it might be due to congestion in the liver or even stones. Such substances in the liver put pressure on it, causing it to make smaller amounts of bile. Less bile means less cholesterol is shuttled out of the body, because that's what bile does. Think about your liver as you might think about your garden hose. What if it had a kink in it? Much less water would squirt through. So if you take a drug to lower your cholesterol level, is that going to solve the real problem? Consider trying a liver cleanse to see what happens.

Symptoms of a sluggish liver

How do you know if you have liver toxicity? There isn't a test as such to determine your status. Only extreme liver damage shows up on a test. Many people think they have a healthy liver because their liver enzymes in blood tests seem normal, but that may be because these enzymes are elevated only when there is advanced liver damage with conditions such as cirrhosis of the liver, liver inflammation, or hepatitis. Therefore, the best thing you can do to tell if you need a liver cleanse is to look at symptoms. But even if you have none of the symptoms, it's still a very good idea to do a liver cleanse at least once a year.

Check off the box next to any symptoms you are experiencing. I recommend you complete a liver cleanse if you have even a few of these symptoms listed below:[4]

☐ Abdominal discomfort

☐ Aches or pains

☐ Allergies

☐ Anal itching (may be a sign of parasites)

☐ Bad breath

☐ Body odor

☐ Brown spots on the face and/or hands

☐ Candidiasis

☐ Cellulite

☐ Constipation

☐ Dark circles under eyes

☐ Digestive problems (belching and/or flatulence)

☐ Dizziness

☐ Drowsiness after eating

☐ Fatigue

☐ Frequent urination at night

☐ Hemorrhoids

☐ Low heat or cold tolerance

☐ Irritability

☐ Loss of memory or inability to concentrate

☐ Loss of sexual desire

☐ Lower back pain

☐ Malaise

☐ Menstrual problems

☐ Migraine headaches or headaches that involve a feeling of fullness or heaviness

☐ Nasal itching (may also be a sign of parasites)

☐ Nervousness and anxiety

☐ Pain around the right shoulder blade and shoulder (also connected with gallbladder congestion)

☐ Premenstrual syndrome

☐ Puffy eyes and/or face

☐ Red nose

☐ Sallow or jaundiced complexion

☐ Sinus problems

☐ Sleeplessness (insomnia)

☐ Small red spots on the skin (either smooth or raised and hard—known as cherry angiomas)

☐ Whitish or yellow tongue coating (may also be a sign of candidiasis or spleen congestion)

Raw soups to the rescue!

If you have a few or more of these symptoms, it's time to begin a liver cleanse. Are you ready for true prevention? You can start with the gentle soup detox program. Loaded with antioxidants such as vitamin C, vitamin E, and beta-carotene, these nutrient heroes will help you detoxify safely.

Eating liver-friendly vegetables will supply the antioxidants that help to bind up free radicals released in the detoxification process. Here is a list of vegetables you should consume during the cleanse:[5]

- Artichokes
- Beets
- Broccoli

- Kale
- Kohlrabi
- Lettuce

- Brussels sprouts
- Cabbage
- Carrots
- Cauliflower
- Celery
- Chives
- Cucumber
- Eggplant
- Garlic
- Green beans

- Mustard greens
- Okra
- Onion
- Parsley
- Parsnips
- Peas
- Pumpkin
- Spinach
- Squash
- Sweet potatoes and yams

Juice, blend into raw soups, incorporate into cooked soups, and eat an abundance of these liver-friendly vegetables during your liver-detoxification program.

A few vegetables in particular to eat in your soups are beets, carrots, and dark leafy greens. Beets have been used in naturopathic medicine to cleanse and support the liver. Beet juice, made with the root and the leaves, is an integral part of my seven-day liver-cleansing program. Carrots help stimulate and improve overall liver function. Dark leafy greens are rich in chlorophyll—a pigment that gives plants their lovely green color. It's essential for photosynthesis, which is the process by which plants absorb energy from light. Greens are vital plants that help detoxify the liver and the blood, literally scavenging toxins from the bloodstream. They are also good yeast killers. Greens also will help to cleanse away heavy metals, chemicals, and pesticides. And they help improve bile flow. All greens are good, so choose whatever you like and try some new ones too. For soup recipes utilizing greens, carrots, and beets, see chapter 8.

To aid the detoxification process, it is also best to avoid meat, dairy, sweets, alcohol, eggs, refined foods, fried foods, sodas, all oils and spreads except olive oil and coconut oil, coffee, and all nonorganic and GMO foods.

Liver-cleanse menu plan

For seven consecutive days, eat at least three raw soups that incorporate many of the liver-friendly vegetables listed. You can have more than three per day, but you should not have less. (You can substitute some of the soups for fresh vegetable juices.)

Also include the following in your plan:

- Water. Drink at least eight glasses of water a day.

- Milk thistle. This herb is known to protect the liver. Its active ingredient silymarin prevents free-radical damage in the liver. It's an excellent liver support herb. You may add this to your soups.

- Artichoke powder. This is very helpful in aiding liver cleansing due to the substance that gives artichokes a bitter taste.

If you'd like to increase bile production and strengthen the bile duct, artichoke powder is your supplement. It is known to break up fat that has been stored in the liver and is helpful to lower cholesterol. This also can be added to your soups.

- Turmeric, a member of the ginger family, is an anti-inflammatory spice that is known to detoxify the liver. Curcumin is a phytonutrient that gives turmeric its bright yellow color. According to the University of Maryland Medical Center curcumin can encourage bile production within the gallbladder. This bile is used within the liver to help remove toxins from the body as well as rejuvenate the liver. Because of this, turmeric has been accepted by some as a treatment for digestion and liver disorders. This spice can help you detox and prevent diseases such as cancer. Turmeric is also a blood purifier, and it helps digestion and elimination. You can get fresh turmeric and blend it into raw soups or you can juice it or just use the powdered spice in your soup.[6]

- Beet greens can be blended easily into your raw soup as they are known to detoxify the liver. They are also very helpful in balancing pH and in improving fat and carbohydrate metabolism. They can also help to lower your cholesterol.

- Black radish, if you can find it, can be blended into your raw soup. You can benefit from its nutrients that help cleanse heavy metals from your liver.

- Dandelion is known to be a liver detoxifier. It encourages bile secretion and promotes waste elimination. You can make dandelion juice or raw soup.

- Garlic is a good source of allicin, which is its active ingredient, and selenium. Both of these compounds are helpful for cleansing the liver. You can add garlic to just about any soup recipe.

Benefits of cleansing the liver

Here are some of the benefits you could receive from completing a liver cleansing:

- Brighter and clearer complexion

- Fading of dark circles under eyes

- Improvement of age spots

- Improved digestion

- Easier weight loss

- Improved and removed cellulite

- More energy

- Easier and more restful sleep

- Fewer aches and pains

- Fewer or less severe headaches

- Improved memory

- Feeling a sense of well-being

- Less severe or fewer allergy symptoms

- Less facial puffiness

- No more anal and nasal itching

- Less body odor

- No coating on tongue

- Less nighttime urination

- Improved sexual desire

- Lessening of back pain

- Less nervousness, anxiety, and restlessness

- Facial redness going away

- Improved sinus problems

- Fewer PMS symptoms

Liver-cleansing recipes

LIVER-CLEANSING RAW BEET SOUP

1 medium raw beet, scrubbed and cut into chunks
½ ripe avocado, peeled and cut into chunks
½ small onion, finely chopped
2–3 fresh dill sprigs
¼ cup fresh parsley
1 tsp. raw apple cider
1 tsp. coconut aminos or tamari
1 cup purified water
2–3 Tbsp. lime juice (1 lime)
¼ tsp. sea salt
Freshly ground black pepper

Blend all ingredients until smooth and enjoy! Serves 1.

GREEN DETOX SOUP IN THE RAW

3 kale leaves, roughly chopped
1 fennel bulb, finely diced
1 cup fresh spinach
2 ribs celery, roughly chopped
2–3 Tbsp. lime juice (1 lime)
½ cup unsweetened coconut milk
1 avocado
1 green organic apple (optional)

Blend all ingredients until smooth. Enjoy! Serves 1.

LYMPHATIC SYSTEM
SOUPER CLEANSE

The lymphatics are your garbage collection system, which is made up of glands, lymph nodes, thymus gland, spleen, and tonsils. Without this system working up to speed, your cells will not get cleansed properly. A colorless fluid called lymph grabs waste and toxins and dumps them in lymph nodes and glands so they can be filtered and removed. This system contains white blood cells—our first line of defense. You'll also find fluids, toxins, waste, and fat in the lymph system that is being shuttled off to the liver and kidneys where they can then be eliminated.

Have you ever wondered why so many people with cancer have cancer in their lymph nodes? It is very important to cleanse the lymphatic system of toxins so you can fight disease. But there's one challenge when it comes to accomplishing this. This system does not have a pump like the circulatory system, which has the heart. Instead it relies on exercise to keep it moving and not get congested. And here's a second challenge—most of us live a sedentary lifestyle. This means that lymphatic fluids will stagnate if you don't do something about it. It's like having clogged pipes in your bathroom. You need to keep these fluids moving through your pipes.

There are a few ways to accomplish this. Exercise more or get a specialized massage called lymphatic drainage massage. You may also do a lymphatic system cleanse that would include the lymph node cleanse soup (see below) and a tincture for lymphatics. (See the appendix.)

I also recommend a machine called a lymphasizer. It's a unit that moves the body like a fish moves through water. Lie on the floor with your feet in the grooves. Set it for ten to twenty minutes, and it will gently rock your body and move your lymphatic system. I love my machine. I use it often, and I know it works. When lymph leaves your body in more significant amounts, it looks like soapy bubbles (not cloudy or frothy, which can indicate kidney problems) in your urine so don't be alarmed if your lymph system is cleansing. (See the appendix for the lymphasizer information.)

Symptoms of lymphatic system congestion

Here are symptoms of lymphatic system congestion:

☐ Swollen fingers and eyes

☐ Puffy face

☐ Sore and stiff body, primarily in the morning

☐ Fatigue

☐ Bloating

☐ Itchiness

☐ Breast swelling or soreness (with your cycle)

☐ Dry skin

☐ Brain fog

☐ Cold hands and feet

If you have one or more of these symptoms, consider doing a lymph cleanse.

Lymph cleanse

Make sure to include foods that will help stimulate the activity of your lymphatic system in your soups and smoothies during a lymph cleanse. These foods include the following:

- Lemon
- Berries
- Greens
- Sunflower seeds
- Pumpkin seeds
- Chia seeds
- Hemp seeds
- Flax seeds
- Herbs and spices
- Seaweed and algae
- Beets

Lymphatic system soup cleanse menu plan

An effective lymphatic system cleanse should last for three to seven days. For the duration, eat as much of the Lymph Node Detoxifying Soup (recipe below) as you like. You may eat other soups, but you should have at least two servings of this soup. Drink at least eight glasses of purified water each day. You may have as much herbal tea as you like. You can have two low-sugar fruits such as berries, a green apple, or a pear between soup meals. Do not eat other foods during this cleanse.

LYMPH NODE DETOX SOUP

This is an excellent recipe for anyone battling cancer that has impacted their lymph nodes. It is also great for anyone who wants prevention, detoxification, and healing.

    1 onion, chopped
    1 small head of green cabbage, chopped
    2 garlic cloves, minced
    2 carrots, chopped
    2 ribs celery, chopped
    1 bunch parsley, chopped
    4 kale leaves, chopped
    2 Nori sheets
    1 cup brown rice
    2 quarts purified water
    Coconut aminos or Bragg's Aminos to taste

In a large stockpot combine all ingredients. Simmer for 1½ hours, then serve. Serves 2.

HAPPY CLEANSING!

I hope you will enjoy these soup-cleansing programs and add some of the other detox protocols to your cleanse. (More cleanse plans are available on my website. See the appendix.) The detox plans and protocols listed in this book will make a difference in how you feel. It can prevent serious diseases down the road, and it can change your life.

CHAPTER 5

A "SOUPER" WEIGHT-LOSS SOLUTION

*Soup puts the heart at ease, calms
down the violence of hunger,
eliminates the tension of the day, and
awakens and refines the appetite.*[1]

—AUGUSTE ESCOFFIER

RECENTLY HEARD A story about Catherine, a woman who spent years of her life and thousands of dollars trying to lose weight. Despite her best intentions, the excess pounds refused to come off, something many of us have experienced. Similar to many other women, Catherine tried all the usual weight-loss regimes. However, even though the weight-loss strategies changed, the results never did: she would lose a few pounds and then gain more back.

Catherine's frustrations came to a head while getting ready to attend a friend's wedding. "Despite all the excitement leading up to the wedding," Catherine shared, "whenever I looked in the mirror, I just wanted to cry.... Obviously I needed to lose a substantial amount of weight, and I needed to lose it quickly. But based on past experience, I didn't like my chances."[2]

Most people in Catherine's shoes would have turned to the plethora of products put out by the dieting industry. But Catherine had already gone down that road and knew such products didn't work. This time she needed to try something completely different. In desperation Catherine turned to a protocol that almost seems too simple to work: she began eating soup—cabbage soup.

A week later, by the day of the wedding, Catherine had lost eleven pounds.

Catherine's story challenges us to rethink some of the things we've been told about weight loss. What if the solution to weight loss is as simple as a bowl of soup?

SOUP RESEARCH

In this chapter we will take a journey through some exciting research about the relationship between soup and weight loss. Here is a smattering of some of the research relating to soup and weight loss:

- A study published in 2013 looked at the effect of eating soup in a sample of 4,158 adults from age nineteen to sixty-four. The study found that people who regularly eat soup are less likely to be overweight.[3]

- A study published in *Appetite* in November 2007 found that those who start off their meals with soup will likely eat less during the actual meal.[4]

- In 2009 BBC News ran a story on "dieting's best kept secret."[5] They reported that eating various foods in soup helps control the appetite and therefore helps promote weight loss significantly more than eating those same foods individually.[6]

- In January 2005 the journal *Physiology & Behavior* published the results of a study conducted on thirteen men and eighteen women. They found that eating soup decreased the amount of calories the subjects consumed throughout the day.[7]

- In June 2005 the journal *Obesity* reported the results of a yearlong clinical trial that showed that eating low calorie-dense soup twice a day led to nearly 50 percent more weight loss than eating two energy-dense snack foods.[8] Research conducted with children at Pennsylvania State University discovered a number of benefits associated with large servings of vegetable soup at the start of the meal. In the group given the soup, the overall intake of calories was reduced while positively influencing children's vegetable consumption.[9]

SOUP IT UP BEFORE YOUR MEAL

Many people avoid eating a soup as a starter before a meal out of a desire to limit overall food consumption. But while the desire to limit calorie intake is good, skipping the soup starter may not be the best way to limit food consumption. It may seem counterintuitive, but the research actually shows that eating soup before a meal helps a person want to eat less during the main meal.

In a 2007 study a group of average-weight adults were given low-calorie soup before lunch once a week for five weeks. After eating the soup, they were given their main meal. Another group was given the same meal but without the soup starter. Most of us would expect that the group that was given more food would end up eating more, but the researchers found that that was actually the opposite. The group that was offered soup before their meal consumed 20 percent fewer calories at that meal. The amazing thing is that this total calorie count included the soup. Those who ate soup before their meals ate fewer calories overall.[10]

Other studies have confirmed the link between eating soup and calorie reduction. For example, a 2005 study conducted with thirty-one subjects discovered that eating soup "led to reductions of hunger and increases of fullness that were comparable to the solid foods."[11] Moreover, "daily energy [calorie] intake tended to be lower on days of soup ingestion compared to the solid foods."[12]

Try it yourself. Begin treating yourself to a soup starter before your meal. This will encourage you to eat less, and it won't require you to muster tons of willpower. When you are eating out, get a soup instead of an appetizer for the same reason. When ordering Chinese food, wonton soup and egg drop soup are relatively nutritious options, especially when compared to other appetizers. If the soup is served with a bread bowl, you can avoid hundreds of calories by not eating the bread. Avoid soup toppings such as croutons, cheese, and sour cream for the same reason.

For maximum benefit you should eat soup about thirty minutes prior to the main meal. This thirty-minute period gives your stomach and brain the chance to register what you have eaten. Consequently, when you sit down for your main course, your hunger will already be partially satiated. This provides two benefits: it will be easier to eat smaller portions during the main meal and you will be less inclined to crave calorie-rich foods during the meal.

Although every person's body responds differently, in general a person will need to reduce her calorie intake by five hundred calories a day to lose a pound a week. This can be accomplished by eating less, but exercising more is also an option. Your best option is to do both, and soup can play an important role in this process by satiating your appetite prior to a main meal.

The soup starter will be even more effective if you combine it with these additional measures:

- Replace starchy foods, such as rice or potatoes, with low-starch vegetables.

- Drink water instead of soda and fruit juice.

- Prepare your foods using only good fats and no sugar, and when you do cook with fats, focus on fats that are healthy fats, such as virgin olive oil, coconut oil, and grapeseed oil.

- Don't snack between meals.

- Shoot for 1,200–1,500 calories total per day for the average woman (1,200 calories is the absolute lowest you should go), although this number can vary a great deal depending on how much exercise you are getting as well as your overall body mass.

Soup Science

In 1999 the *American Journal of Clinical Nutrition* published fascinating research conducted on three groups of lean women at Pennsylvania State University. These women consumed breakfast, lunch, and dinner in the laboratory once per week for four weeks. On three of those days several minutes before the main meal, the women were given a starter consisting of chicken rice casserole, chicken rice casserole and a glass of water, or a chicken rice soup containing the same ingredients (type and amount) as the casserole that was served with water. After consuming these preloads, the women were free to choose whatever they fancied for lunch. Interestingly after the women were given soup, they consumed significantly fewer calories at lunchtime.[13]

We have seen that soup is effective in satiating appetite, which helps a person limit overall consumption, but why is this? The answer is not simply that soup simply has healthy low-calorie ingredients. As we have seen in several studies, if you were to take the ingredients that go into a typical soup and eat those ingredients separately, while also drinking the same amount of water that would be in the soup, it won't satiate your appetite as soup will. The feeling of fullness will last only a couple hours at most. On the other hand, if you take those same ingredients and blend them with water to make a soup, your hunger will be abated for much longer, thus discouraging snacking in the interval between meals.

To uncover the secrets for why blending food into soup makes such a difference, we have to understand some of the science behind what occurs in the stomach. Science author Jack Challoner explained for the BBC what researchers discovered about how soup interacts with the digestive juices in the stomach:

> Scientists have used ultrasound and MRI scans of people's stomachs to investigate what happens after eating solid-food-plus-water meals compared with the same food made into soup.
>
> After you eat a meal, the pyloric sphincter valve at the bottom of your stomach holds food back so that the digestive juices can get to work. Water, however, passes straight through the sphincter to your intestines, so drinking water does not contribute to "filling you up."
>
> When you eat the same meal as a soup, the whole mixture remains in the stomach, because the water and food are blended together.... The stomach stays fuller for longer, staving off those hunger pangs.[14]

I hope it is beginning to make sense why a soup starter (especially when consumed half an hour before the main meal) can play a crucial role in limiting your food intake. This is especially true of soups that are high in fiber and protein since these ingredients are filling but don't add a lot of calories.

SOUPER SLOW

Another benefit to including soup in your meals is that it forces you to slow down. Given the process of eating soup with a spoon out of a bowl one bite at a time, it is difficult to rush consuming soup. If you sip your soup with a teaspoon instead of a soup spoon, it will take even longer. Slow eating has been linked to a number of benefits, including helping people to voluntarily reduce their calorie intake.[15] Moreover, the time involved in eating soup gives your brain opportunity to register fullness.

THE TRUTH ABOUT SOUP
AND WEIGHT LOSS

Did you know it's possible to lose weight without being hungry all the time?

Many people erroneously think that to lose weight you have to be perpetually hungry. Nothing could be further from the truth. To lose weight properly, it is more important to pay attention to what you eat than how you eat. In particular the goal should be to eat the most nutrient-dense food you can get. We say a food has nutrient density when it provides more nutrients for fewer calories.

Most soups have a rich nutrient content. They tend to be low in calories; limited in fats, sugars, and processed starches; and high in the nutrients your body needs to stay fit and healthy.

SOUPER HEALTHY
WEIGHT-LOSS SOLUTIONS!

Not all soups are created equal. Choosing the right type of soup is important for weight loss. The healthiest and most slimming soups are vegetable soups that use a basic broth/stock and a lean protein source (lean meat, fish, or beans/legumes).

Research suggests that pureed vegetable soup and

chunky-pureed vegetable soup are particularly effective in satiating the appetite and therefore useful in the context of a weight-loss program.[16] In fact, dietary guidelines put out by the US Department of Health and Human Services in 2010 reported that individuals who consume broth-based soups may have a better chance at controlling their weight.[17]

Because of how soup increases satiety (that feeling of fullness at the end of a meal), it makes an excellent main dish. Try the following experiment: on two nights a week swap out a normal high-calorie meal for a main dish of soup, and then record how many pounds you lose. For even better results, supplement the soup with a salad instead of bread. Try this for one to three weeks, and the results will speak for themselves! The more weeks you do this, the better the results, and you should be celebrating your good results.

Also experiment with how soup can be substituted for some of your normal meals. For example, instead of beef chili, eat a broth-based bean soup with vegetables. Instead of a large plate of pasta with tomato sauce, eat tomato or minestrone soup. Instead of eating the usual snack food between meals, have some soup. Instead of sipping a warm beverage such as hot chocolate or coffee, sip a mug of warm soup or broth. When you go out to dinner, order a cup of miso soup instead of a drink. I love sipping on a cup of miso soup while I wait for my favorite sushi.

Additionally try experimenting with various soups

based on your different needs. If you are trying to lower your blood pressure or reduce hypertension, research shows that gazpacho soup is particularly effective.[18] If you are suffering from a cold and want to reduce congestion, research shows that chicken soup is one of the best options.[19]

SOUPING FOR SLIMMING

In 2014 the *British Journal of Nutrition* published a study of adults aged nineteen to sixty-four. They showed that soup eaters tend to have overall less body weight and slimmer waists than those who don't eat soup. Moreover, regular soup eaters had better overall eating habits that included fewer calories and fat and more protein, fiber, vitamins, and minerals.[20]

When souping for weight loss, the thing that matters is the calorie content. This means that it is best to avoid soups that are rich in cream, cheese, or pasta. Instead, try low-calorie soups made from chicken, beans, and vegetables such as mushroom, tomato, or carrot.

The "Soup Diet" is easy! All you need to do is to make a large batch of soup, enough to last you for the rest of the week. Every time you make a new soup, freeze a little bit for the busy days when you've run out of soup.

SOUPS TO AVOID

Just because something is called "soup" doesn't make it healthy. When souping-for-slimming, be wary of ready-to-eat soups. Not only are ready-made soups high in calories, but they may also provide more sodium than your body needs. Too much sodium can result in high blood pressure and an increased risk of heart disease. For example, a single can of Campbell's Chunky New England Clam Chowder has 420 calories, 20 grams of fat, and 1,780 milligrams of sodium.[21] Canned soups also contain high levels of BPA, a chemical associated with increased risk of heart disease and diabetes.[22]

To avoid these problems, make soup yourself. By controlling what goes into the soup, you control what goes in your mouth. In the process you will also be controlling the size of your waist.

SOUP AND EXERCISE

Soup is not a magic formula for weight loss, especially if you are not prepared to make lifestyle changes. In particular it is important that you exercise. The combination of soup plus exercise is a very effective way to manage your weight long-term. Exercise boosts your metabolism, enabling you to burn fat even when you are resting.

WEIGHT-LOSS SOUPS

Cabbage soup diet

The cabbage soup diet is popular in the weight-loss community for short-term slimming. It is a form of fasting that offers your body a chance to detox as well as lose weight.

Cabbage is a superfood chock-full of vitamin C, fiber, antioxidants, vitamin K, protein, and many other amazing nutrients. Even better, cabbage digests slowly. From a weight-loss perspective, any food that digests slowly is a bonus since it helps you feel full longer. When you feel full, you are less likely to crave other food.

While this diet is not recommended for long-term weight management, it can be particularly effective for short-term slimming, as we saw with Catherine's story at the beginning of this chapter. To follow this diet, have a juice or raw soup for breakfast with one serving of protein, such as a boiled egg or some nuts. For the rest of the day, just eat cabbage soup. For a delicious cabbage soup recipe, see chapter 8.

Chicken soup diet

Many weight-loss diets leave you feeling perpetually hungry. Not so on the chicken soup diet. This seven-day diet allows you to eat breakfast each day followed by as much chicken soup as you desire. Breakfast can be vegetable juice, a green smoothie, or eggs and whole-grain toast. After breakfast, no food except chicken soup and a side salad is consumed until the next morning. An olive-oil-based dressing is allowed with the salad. Get your chicken soup recipes in chapter 8.

Cherie's watercress soup diet

See chapter 8 for the Sweet Watercress Soup and Watercress Detox Soup recipes. Here's the diet plan for the week:

Day 1

- Treat yourself to as much watercress soup as you fancy.

- Eat as much fruit as you like from the fruit list below. (If you are sensitive to fruit or you have diabetes or hypoglycemia and must limit fruit, choose from the vegetable list, also below.)

Day 2

- Continue to eat as much watercress soup as you like.

- Eat as many vegetables as you want from the list of approved vegetables.

Day 3

- Eat as much watercress soup as you like.

- Choose one to two servings food from the fruit list.

- Choose at least five to six servings from the vegetable list.

Day 4

- Follow the same plan as day one.

Day 5

- Eat as much watercress soup as you like.

- Eat fish and skinless, lean chicken. Only eat as much as necessary to satisfy hunger.

- Eat fresh tomatoes.

Day 6

- Follow the same as plan as day five, but in addition eat anything on the vegetable list.

Day 7

- Eat as much watercress soup as you like.

- Eat anything on the fruit list.

- Eat anything on the vegetable list.

As an alternative, you can follow the plan below, which is simplified.

Start your day with 1 cup of hot water with lemon juice and a dash of cayenne. This will get your liver moving, which is important for a good metabolism.

Two of your meals each day should be Watercress Detox Soup or Sweet Watercress Soup. (Recipes for both soups can be found in chapter 8.) You can eat as much soup as you like. The third meal should be a low-carb meal, such as a main course salad with protein (chicken, turkey, or fish). Other options include veggies and protein, such as steamed asparagus and baked chicken or grilled salmon; a stir-fry of vegetables and meat; or a breakfast of eggs and vegetables.

Watercress Soup Diet Vegetable List[23]

Artichoke	Eggplant
Asparagus	Lettuce
Beans	Mushrooms
Beetroot	Onions
Broccoli	Parsley
Brussels sprouts	Peppers
Cabbage	Radishes
Carrots	Spinach
Cauliflower	Turnip
Celery	Watercress
Cucumber	Zucchini

Diet Fruit List[24]

Apples	Nectarines
Apricots	Oranges
Blueberries	Peaches
Cherries	Pineapple
Grapefruit	Plums
Grapes	Raspberries
Kiwi	Strawberries
Lemons	Tangerines
Melons	

SOUP IT UP WITH FOODS THAT HELP YOU LOSE WEIGHT

The good thing about soup is that there are no rules—you can add in anything you like. Here are some foods you can routinely add to your soups to maximize the opportunities for weight loss:

- Mushrooms: The rich, meaty taste of mushrooms make them a perfect substitute for meat. A yearlong study showed that swapping out red meat for white button mushrooms leads to weight loss.[25]

- Legumes: Studies have shown that eating four servings of legumes per week as part of a calorie-restricted diet improves weight loss more effectively than an equivalent diet not that does not include them.[26]

- Watercress: The good thing about watercress is that it provides nutrients without significant addition of calories. Considered a superfood, this aquatic plant is one of the most nutrient-dense vegetables known to man.

- Almonds: A study of sixty-five overweight adults who were on a calorie-restricted diet found that eating a quarter cup of almonds decreased weight more effectively than a snack comprised of complex carbohydrates. After twenty-four weeks those who ate almonds experienced a 62 percent greater reduction in weight.[27]

- Coconut oil: Not all fat is bad. In fact, coconut oil is positively good for you and helps you lose weight. The liver prefers burning for fuel the medium-chain triglycerides in coconut oil. The high concentration of medium-chain triglycerides in coconut oil causes it to boost satiety compared to other fats, in addition to helping to burn off excess body fat. The additional benefits of coconut oil are too numerous to relate here and could be the topic of an entire chapter in itself.

THERMOGENIC FOODS THAT REV UP YOUR METABOLISM

Thermogenic foods are those that produce heat in the body. Heat raises metabolism and thus burns calories. A 2010 study of animals found that obesity occurred when animals "didn't produce enough heat after eating, not because the animals ate more or were less active."[28] It should be a no-brainer that if you are trying to lose weight, you need plenty of thermogenic foods to help you burn fat. You can easily add many of these foods to your soups for an extra kick.

- Hot peppers: When you include hot peppers in your soup, you increase your metabolism and burn more calories.[29]

- Garlic: In a 2011 study published in the *Journal of Nutrition*, researchers fed obese mice either a garlic supplement or a placebo for several weeks. The mice given garlic had a higher body temperature and lost body weight and fat, and those on the placebo did not experience this. The higher body temperature of the mice on the garlic supplement indicated a thermogenic effect–promoted weight loss.[30]

- Ginger: According to a study in *Metabolism*, "ginger has a thermogenic effect by enhancing the thermic effect of food as well as promoting feelings of satiety."[31] Ginger really sparks up your soup recipe with lovely spicy flavor.

- Black pepper: This spice contains an active compound known as piperine that gives pepper its flavor. This compound "has been shown to help the body burn more calories and can also help your body use nutrients more efficiently."[32] It also encourages a metabolic reaction that helps to break down fat cells. Use freshly ground pepper to get the most piperine, the compound that has the greatest effect on fat and weight loss.[33]

NO MORE DIET BLUES

For many of us, even the term *weight loss* has become associated with unpleasant diets and miserable lifestyles. However much we may want to shed unwanted pounds, the very thought of starting another weight-loss program may fill us with dread. As we've seen in this chapter, there is a simple solution to this problem. All you need to do is begin making your own soup. By simply having tasty soup on hand for when you need to satisfy your hunger cravings and by eating a bowl of soup before your main meal, you increase your chances of losing weight without ever having to muster up tons of willpower or face the diet blues. Then if you want to accelerate your weight loss, you can do a soup diet for one or more days in a row and watch the pounds fly away.

CHAPTER 6

THE HEALING
POWER OF SOUP

*The lore has not died out of the
world, and you will still find people
who believe that soup will cure any
hurt or illness and is no bad thing
to have for the funeral either.*[1]
—JOHN STEINBECK

WHEN I WAS a little girl, my grandmother's answer
for nearly every illness was a big pot of chicken
soup. We had a lot of that soup because I was sick all
the time. It is still my go-to food when my husband or
I catch a bug. But there's a lot more to soup than just a
cup of healing elixir when you're sick. Soup can help you
lose weight, as we already discussed, and it can keep you
from getting sick. I'm excited to share with you all the
wonderful benefits that are available in a bowl of soup.

VEGGIE FEVER

First off, soup is a great way to eat more vegetables. It can give you an advantage in trying to meet your daily recommended number of servings of vegetables. You can add a variety of vegetables, and since they are masked in the soup flavors, you can even add vegetables you don't particularly like. You'll hardly know they are there; just dice them up into small pieces. Also, for really picky eaters who may turn up their noses at anything green, you can puree some green vegetables and then pour the mixture into the soup pot. A "Dutch study showed that when healthy toddlers were given vegetable soups containing endive and spinach twice a week over a seven-week period, there was a marked difference in the acceptance compared to those who didn't undergo the soup exposure."[2]

While raw vegetables play an important role in the human diet, some veggies pack a bigger nutritional punch when cooked. The cooking process helps to break down resilient cell walls, making nutrients easier to absorb. For example, fresh tomatoes can provide us only a fraction of their available lycopene, while cooked portions give our bodies a large dose of the powerful antioxidant. Similarly, the absorbable amount of beta-carotene, precursor to vitamin A, is increased by cooking carrots and squashes such as pumpkin and butternut squash. Asparagus is another veggie that can be persuaded to release more nutrients by the application of heat, in this case essential vitamins A, C, and E.[3]

One drawback to cooking vegetables is that some of the water-soluble vitamins are lost when the cooking water is tossed out. Soups are the perfect solution to this problem because these vitamins and minerals end up in the tasty broth. Another advantage of cooking veggies in soups can be found with the addition of leafy greens such as spinach or kale. Since greens decrease so much in volume when cooked, you can add an entire bunch of spinach and end up with a high concentration of folate in your bowl!

VEGETABLE SOUP CAN FIGHT CELL DAMAGE

After a study conducted at Tufts University in Boston, researchers reported that those eating gazpacho twice a day had lower stress levels as indicated by blood tests after only seven days. "The researchers say the beneficial effect was due at least in part to an increase in vitamin C intake."[4] The study asked the twelve participants to continue their normal diet and lifestyle with one important difference: they consumed 17 ounces of gazpacho each day for fourteen days. Rich in vitamin C, gazpacho is a cold, Spanish soup made from fresh tomatoes that are crushed in a blender along with raw peppers, onions, cucumbers, garlic, oil, and spices. Blood samples collected at the end of the first and second weeks of the study showed elevated levels of vitamin C in all the participants, a 26 percent increase for the men and 25 percent for the women. Vitamin C has powerful antioxidant properties that reduce cell damage caused by free radicals; however, the results of the study indicated that more was going on.[5]

Antonio Martin, the study's lead investigator, said the functions of vitamin C at the molecular level "include a major role in preventing the formation of compounds involved in abnormal inflammation and a biochemical process called oxidative stress, both of which can alter cells in ways that set the stage for chronic diseases."[6] While these antioxidant and anti-inflammatory benefits can be obtained by eating foods other than soups, the researchers suspected that the unique combination of vegetables contained in the gazpacho may have produced a collaborative force.[7]

After just seven days of eating gazpacho, the volunteers had a significant reduction in prostaglandin E2, a stress molecule that is found when inflammation is present in the body. These same blood samples also showed lower concentrations of other stress markers, including an isoprostane molecule (prostaglandin-like compound) normally found in higher levels as age increases and also when chronic disease is present. In addition, amounts of monocyte chemotactic protein-1 (inflammatory compound) were reduced. This molecule is found in the types of plaque that clog arteries and lead to heart disease.[8]

Yet another positive finding in the blood samples was a decrease in uric acid levels—an 18 percent reduction for the men and an 8 percent reduction for the women. Ordinarily the kidneys clean uric acid from the blood, but when high levels accumulate in the body, uric acid forms sharp crystals that collect around the joints, causing inflammation and the painful condition known as gout. Uric acid may also weaken cells that line the blood vessels, which can lead to heart disease.[9]

As the vitamin C concentrations increased, there was a direct, inverse proportion of the mentioned compounds that typically lead to negative health conditions. The researchers believe the correlation suggests that the vitamin C protected against the damaging effects of oxidative stress and inflammation. That's a potent bowl of gazpacho!

JET FUEL FOR YOUR IMMUNE SYSTEM

Could soup actually improve the workings of the body's immune system? The immune system consists of organs, tissues, and cells that fight off pathogenic organisms and substances that can do us harm, and while many of our lifestyle choices can support immune function—adequate sleep, physical activity, stress management—good nutrition tops the list. Preparing a delicious pot of soup or blending up a yummy raw soup presents the opportunity to combine superfoods into a medley our immune system will thank us for.

Antioxidants are the immune system's best nutritional ally, and vegetables are one of the best sources. Besides slowing the aging process and neutralizing free radicals, some unique antioxidants in vegetables actually repair damaged molecules, provide a shield effect for your DNA, and even cause some cancer cells to destroy themselves. Whether chopped, shredded, blended, or pureed, pretty much any variety of veggie you have on hand can come to the party!

No immune-boosting arsenal is complete without legumes. Adding dried peas, beans, or lentils to your soup will transform it into a hearty meal complete with protein and lots of filling, water-soluble fiber. In general the regular consumption of any type of legume can lead to health benefits such as lowering cholesterol, blood pressure, and inflammation. They enhance immunity and provide protection from cancer.

The woodsy flavor of mushrooms makes a great addition to a bowl of soup, but the nutritional value is also hard to beat. Mushrooms have been discovered to contain profound medicinal properties. "Long chain polysaccharides, particularly alpha and beta glucan molecules, are primarily responsible for the mushrooms' beneficial effect on your immune system. In one study, adding one or two servings of dried shiitake mushrooms was found to have a beneficial, modulating effect on immune system function. Another study done on mice found that white button mushrooms enhanced the adaptive immunity response to salmonella."[10]

Make your soup something special with the distinctive taste of garlic, ginger, or turmeric—bonus points for using all three! Garlic, onions, leeks, and shallots are known for their pungent aroma, but they also spark the production of glutathione, an antioxidant that helps to eliminate toxins and carcinogens. Sharp and spicy, ginger mellows in flavor when cooked for longer periods, such as the slow simmer required for some soups. Ginger contains gingerol, a substance with both antioxidant and anti-inflammatory properties. Turmeric and its yellow ingredient curcumin have another impressive anti-inflammatory and antioxidant effect. Curcumin is poorly absorbed on its own, but this is remedied by consuming black pepper along with turmeric. If you are blending fresh turmeric in a raw soup, add a dash of pepper.

CHICKEN SOUP FIGHTS COLDS AND FLU

Jack Canfield and Mark Victor Hansen enjoyed wild success from their Chicken Soup for the Soul books. Their book sales couldn't have been possible without the general consensus that chicken soup somehow equals healing. But is it true?

In-depth research led by pulmonary expert Dr. Stephen Rennard demonstrated the healing power of chicken soup. In his lab at the University of Nebraska Medical Center, Dr. Rennard found evidence that chicken soup has anti-inflammatory characteristics that can prevent cold symptoms. He tested blood samples from volunteers who consumed an old family chicken soup recipe and discovered that white blood cells formed by the presence of a viral cold infection did not migrate to the lung area as they usually do. He pointed to an unknown ingredient in the chicken soup that blocked or slowed the movement of the infection-fighting cells, theorizing that less mucus would form as a result. The tested recipe came from a Lithuanian grandmother on his wife's side of the family and contained chicken, onions, sweet potatoes, parsnips, turnips, carrots, celery, parsley, salt, and pepper. "The biologically active material is unknown," Rennard said. "It may be that some complex chemistry takes place, that the entire concoction makes it work."[11]

Another study held at Mount Sinai in Miami compared the results of drinking cold water, hot water, and chicken soup. Researchers studied how the different liquids affected mucus and air flow in the noses of the volunteers. Both the hot water and soup helped move the nasal mucus, but between the two, the chicken soup had a superior outcome.[12]

QUELL INFLAMMATION

Everyone can identify with the pain of inflammation brought on by an injury or a condition such as arthritis. The pain can be traced back to an enzyme called cyclooxygenase-2, or Cox-2 for short. Cox-2 aids in the production of prostaglandins instrumental in causing inflammation and its resulting pain. Though this is the body's way of fighting off infection and injury, the pain can leave us reaching for medicines that inhibit Cox-2, but they carry side effects with long-term use.

To compound the issue, poor dietary choices can actually cause the body to overproduce Cox-2, resulting in chronic, systemic inflammation. "Too much Cox-2 appears to result from imbalances and deficiencies of certain nutrients. Rather than correct these underlying dietary problems, pharmaceutical Cox-2 inhibitors only mask the most visible symptoms. Relatively minor dietary changes, plus some vitamin and herbal supplements, correct the underlying problems."[13] Tame inflammation the natural way by adding some of the following anti-inflammatory herbs and spices to your next soup recipe.

- Ginger: Known for its ability to remedy digestive trouble, the gingerol in this spicy rhizome can put up a mighty fight against inflammation. "Besides pain relief from arthritis, results of a double-blind comparative clinical trial indicated that ginger (250-mg capsules) was as effective as the non-steroidal anti-inflammatory drugs mefenamic acid (250 mg) and ibuprofen (400 mg) in relieving pain in women with primary dysmenorrhea."[14]

- Turmeric: Turmeric has been used for centuries as both a spice and for healing infections and digestive upset. Curcumin is the active compound in turmeric that gives it its characteristic yellow color and is an extraordinary antioxidant, neutralizing free radicals in the body. Curcumin is also a natural Cox-2 inhibitor, preventing the formation of prostaglandins that cause inflammation.

- Pepper: A powerful spice, pepper is used the world over as an essential flavor enhancer. Piperine gives pepper its anti-inflammatory properties; these properties are even stronger when combined with turmeric. Crank up the peppery heat with cayenne, another pepper that fights inflammation. Capsaicin, the main compound of cayenne, has been found to provide pain relief when used as a cream, but can also be ingested as a tea or in a soup.

- Celery seed: Wild celery originated in the Mediterranean, where its seeds were esteemed for their medicinal versatility, treating everything from colds and flu to water retention and arthritis. Both celery and its seeds contain a substance called 3-n-butylphthalide, or 3nB, discovered recently by researchers at the University of Chicago Medical Center to have the ability to lower blood pressure. The seeds act as a diuretic, helping to rid the body of excess fluid, which not only lowers blood pressure but also reduces inflammation as well. Celery seed extract is also showing promise as a pain reliever for arthritis, fibromyalgia, and gout.[15]

Other ingredients you can add to pump up the anti-inflammatory effects of your soup include alliums such as onion and garlic, and fresh or dried herbs such as rosemary and oregano.

THE HEALING SOUP DIET FOR CROHN'S DISEASE, COLITIS, AND IBS

Many people with Crohn's disease, colitis, or irritable bowel syndrome (IBS) can't eat raw soups or smoothies or drink fresh juice, even though these foods are very nutritious, because they can trigger a flare-up in their disorder or worsen symptoms. Each person is different, but many people have told me they can't eat raw foods at all. My recommendation is a cooked soup diet—just blended, cooked vegetable soup, for at least a week. This gives your intestinal tract a chance to rest and heal with this diet. As you already know, you aren't going to heal your disease by doing the same things you've always been doing. As your intestinal tract heals, you can slowly introduce raw soups and smoothies and fresh veggie juices.

As you embark on your healing journey, you should baby your digestive tract. That is why you'll want to kick off the first week with just blended veggie soups. Do not include any soup with beans, lentils, or split peas. Avoid all gas-producing foods, which are very hard on an irritated gut. Keep in mind that you may feel a bit worse before you get better. Tiredness and headaches are not uncommon as you detox. But you can feel confident that you are doing the right thing to heal your body.

After your week of eating only cooked, blended vegetable soups, you may add steamed vegetables and fish. The week after that you may add just one 6-ounce glass of fresh vegetable juice to see how you do. Make sure to juice only mild vegetables such as zucchini and carrot or green apple and celery, especially for this first week. If this is tolerated well, then you can stick with this regimen. Your diet should be very simple until you heal. If you do not do well with the juice or even the steamed veggies and fish, you may need to stick with the blended soups for a longer period of time. If you do well, you may be able to add brown rice after a few weeks. However, from here on you should completely avoid alcohol, butter, margarine, oils, carbonated beverages, coffee, black tea, chocolate, dairy, gluten, and fried foods.

Your symptoms have been caused by the standard American diet of grains, dairy, meat, processed foods, and junk food. When you are no longer eating the foods that irritated your gut, you can begin to heal. In one month you could feel like a new person. In a year you could be totally healed, as long you stick to your new simple diet.

THE HEALTH BENEFITS
OF BROTH

No discussion of soup's healing powers would be complete without delving into the many health benefits of broths, especially bone broth. Consumption of bone broth has a rich tradition throughout human history, and the nourishing elixir still appears today in the diets of many cultures across the globe. While the typical American might have succumbed to the convenience of highly processed canned soups in the past, the nutritional importance of "old-fashioned" bone broths has gained a new foothold, resulting in a return to traditional methods. And for those in a hurry, organic bone broth is now available at many supermarkets.

"Traditional cultures wisely practiced nose-to-tail eating and consumed all parts of the animal, including the skin, cartilage, tendons, and other gelatinous cuts of meat. This provided a balanced intake of all the amino acids necessary to build and maintain those same structures in the human body."[16] Bone broths are made by a slow simmer of fish, poultry, lamb, or beef bones and feet. Two hours is long enough to extract the nutrients from fish bones, but the larger bones of beef or lamb should be simmered for twenty-four hours. Bones should be sourced from pasture-raised animals or wild-caught fish to reduce toxins and increase the nutrient content. Start by covering the bones with cold water, and be sure to add a splash of apple cider vinegar. The acid will break down the bones and allow their wealth of minerals to infuse the broth.

One of the reasons bone broth is so nutritious is because of its gelatin content. The gelatin forms when the collagen in the bones and cartilage is broken down. You'll notice the gelatin causes the broth, when it is cooled, to congeal into a consistency similar to Jell-O. Since collagen forms the framework of the human body and makes up about a quarter of its protein, adding extracted collagen (gelatin) to the diet is a great idea, especially for the gut. Gelatin strengthens the mucosal lining of the gut, which is responsible for keeping gut microbes away from the intestinal barrier. In addition, gelatin aids the digestive process by pulling digestive juices to food surfaces. Another component of bone broth, the amino acid glycine, stimulates the production of stomach acid, crucial for good digestion.

These attributes have given bone broth its deserved reputation as a gut healer. In one case, a woman who had been unable to keep down any food or water after gallbladder surgery became dehydrated and desperate. Traditional medicine and modern doctors were unable to help her and, in fact, were only exacerbating her condition. She finally was helped by alternative medicine and bone broth! Beginning with one small sip of chicken broth at a time, she gradually increased the amount and was able to keep it down. Eventually she was able to handle solid foods as her gut health was restored.

Loaded with minerals, bone broth delivers calcium,

copper, iron, magnesium, manganese, phosphorus, potassium, sodium, and zinc. Add to that seventeen amino acids, collagen, chondroitin, and glucosamine, plus the healing power of gelatin. Besides being a powerful gut healer, bone broth can help almost every system of the body, from improving cardiovascular health to strengthening bones and joints. It can even improve mood and sleep. Bone broth provides such a bonanza of nutrition, making it a very healthy base for your next pot of soup. (See chapter 8 for my bone broth recipe.)

JUST WHAT THE DOCTOR ORDERED

Sometimes a big bowl of hot soup is just what the doctor ordered. It's not only comfort food; it's *healing* food. A bubbling pot of soup on the stove fills the house with pleasing aromas and fills our hearts with soothing anticipation.

Soup is easily digested, and with the addition of bone broth, soup heals our guts and improves digestion. Soups provide one of the easiest and most palatable ways to add more vegetables into our diet, and more vegetables mean more vitamins, fiber, and phytonutrients along with more antioxidants and better immunity. Soup provides the opportunity to use a variety of spices and herbs, which are some of the best natural medicines on the planet. As part of a healthy diet and lifestyle, that means less inflammation and therefore less vulnerability to modern diseases such as cardiovascular disease, diabetes, autoimmune diseases, and cancer.

Soup warms our bones and hydrates us at the same time. Raw blended soups can refresh us on a warm day. Smooth and creamy, thick and chunky, or thin enough to slurp from a mug, soup can satisfy any craving while delivering superior nutrition. Simple and quick or complicated with layered flavors, no two pots of soup are ever the same. Neither are blended raw soups. There's really only one question to ask: What kind of soup are you going to make today?

CHAPTER 7

HOW DO I BEGIN?

If you fail to plan, you are
planning to fail![1]

—BENJAMIN FRANKLIN

SINCE I WANT you to be able to make the best and healthiest soup possible, I've put together several sections to help you plan ahead for soup making. With it containing everything from tips on tools and equipment to how to choose the healthiest ingredients, this chapter will help you in assembling everything you need to make yummy, healthy soup.

TOOLS AND EQUIPMENT

Having the right equipment can help you make soup an easy process. Here are eight kitchen essentials that can help you turn out and serve great soup creations.

1. Stockpot: The best choice for making soup is an 8-quart stockpot with a heavy

bottom, which will help prevent scorching during long cook times. It should have good gripping handles as well. And if it is a little higher than wide, it will help prevent too much evaporation.

2. Blender or Vitamix: I use my Vitamix often to puree soups for a creamy consistency, but a blender will also work. This is your primary tool for raw blended soups.

3. Hand blender: A hand blender, also commonly called an immersion blender, is all you need to puree butternut squash or potatoes.

4. Food processor: Tired of chopping onions, celery, and carrots? The food processor is a big time saver. Use the pulse function and get your chopped veggies in less than half the time.

5. Long-handled wooden spoon: A well-used wooden spoon is part of the soup tradition in our family. Though you don't have to have one, some people swear it makes soup taste better.

6. Soup ladle: If you get a ladle with a hook on the end, you can rest it over the side of your stock pot.

7. Soup bowls: This seems like a no-brainer unless you go to serve the soup and you don't have them. If you get deep bowls, it will keep your soup warm longer.

8. Glass storage containers: I love my glass containers with snap down lids that give a tight seal. They are great for storing soup in the refrigerator or for freezing it. If you don't have the room in your freezer for many containers, use Ziploc bags.

SAVING TIME BY PREPPING

There are several ways to save time while prepping your soup recipes.

You can save time by doing all your grocery shopping at once. Take your weekly list and plan one (or two) bulk shopping trips. Clean all your produce when you return so you are one step closer to cooking when the time is right.

Then look at your soup recipe and see what ingredients you can prep all at once, in advance, right after you have returned from grocery shopping. For example, you can de-stem all your leafy greens (although that's not necessary when making a raw blended soup), clean them, line them with towels to keep them dry and fresh, and place them in your fridge, ready to chop. You can also mince a head of garlic or a piece of ginger and keep it fresh in your fridge by covering with olive oil. Chop sturdy root vegetables such as carrots, sweet potatoes, and parsnips, and cover them in water in your fridge. Once you start chopping and cleaning produce, you will find you save time by doing a lot at once.

You may want to choose Saturday or Sunday as a soup-making day. Making soup on the weekends is one thing you can do ahead of time to eat well during the week. You can make a big batch of soup and keep it simple.

These are life skills that will benefit your health and relationship with cooking for many years to come.

SPEEDY SOUPS
FOR BUSY DAYS

Even with all the prep work, making soup may some-times seem like a daunting task. When we think of homemade soup, it often brings to mind a simmering pot of soup on the stove top and logging in some serious time at the cutting board. The scarcity of time in our lives temps us to hit the reject button on soup, but pre-paring soup doesn't have to take a lot of time. Before you give up and run for the drive-through, consider one of these quick soup ideas:

- Odds and ends: You know those random veggies at the bottom of your crisper that will likely go to waste? Maybe there's a dab of grilled chicken or the remains of a pot roast at the back of the fridge too. Hopefully you have some bone broth in the freezer, but if not a carton of chicken stock from the pantry will suffice.

Grab a large pot, and turn this into a quick dinner!

- Asian flavor: Frozen vegetables simmered in broth plus some grated ginger and a bit of sesame oil make a great, Asian-flavored soup. You can add some chopped rotisserie chicken from the deli or even drizzle in a couple of beaten eggs for a quick egg drop soup. (A little fish sauce couldn't hurt either.)

- Blended soup: Choose your favorite ingredients and blend them together. Grab a recipe from chapter 8. You can make fruit and veggie raw soups in just minutes. Pour in a glass and take it with you. This is the fastest soup going!

The truth is, soup is one of the easiest, most forgiving meals to prepare. It freezes well and makes the perfect "fast food." Quick soups are economical and nutritious, not to mention a great opportunity to use your creativity and the ingredients in your pantry or refrigerator!

CHOOSE YOUR INGREDIENTS WISELY

For the healthiest, freshest soups, choose ingredients with your health in mind. We discussed earlier how big of a difference living foods make in our lives. That is true for all ingredients, from salt to oils to vegetables and meat.

I'm excited to share guidelines with you for healthy shopping. These are the foods that will energize your body and help you enjoy vibrant health. If you put junk in your body, you'll get a bad return. If you put quality foods in your body, you'll get a great return on your health. It's similar to the fuel you choose for your car. If your car requires premium fuel and you put in regular gasoline, you'll have problems. If you choose diesel and your car wasn't made for it, you'll end up with a dead car.

You were made for premium fuel. In this section you'll discover what that is. Choose organic food whenever possible, and get the freshest produce in season from your farmer's market. This is local farm-to-table fare. When the markets aren't in season, get your organic produce from your local grocery store.

The following is a healthy shopping guide for the best ingredients for your soup.

Salt

I recommend using only true sea salt, Celtic sea salt, pink Himalayan salt, or gray salt. Natural salt is less processed than regular table salt and contains trace minerals and elements that are beneficial to overall health. If you choose the coarse sea salt, you will need a salt mill. I do not recommend Morton's sea salt because it is heavily processed. As with regular table salt, many of the minerals are removed, leaving you primarily with sodium chloride.

Pepper

Purchase whole black peppercorns and grind (or crack) them fresh for each recipe using a pepper mill to get the most piperine. Fresh pepper will help you detoxify your body. And good news for weight loss! The outer layer of the peppercorn helps the body break down fat cells. Pepper is also known to stimulate hydrochloric acid—a plus for digestion.

Cooking oils

Here's the scoop on oils. Ditch safflower, sunflower, soy, corn, and canola oil (canola is made from rapeseed, a big GMO crop). These are polyunsaturated oils that oxidize easily and create free radicals that damage cells and create inflammation.

Following is a list of good oils and their smoke points. If an oil starts to smoke, it is oxidizing; throw it out and start over.

- Almond oil is used for high-heat cooking with a smoke point of 420 degrees.

- Avocado oil has a medium smoke point of 375 to 400 degrees.

- Virgin organic coconut oil is a slimming oil that received unfounded negative reviews for a few decades, which was promoted by the seed and vegetable oil industry to steal market share. This oil is actually heart healthy. It's also delicious.

It has a smoke point of 350 degrees, making it suitable for mid-temperature cooking.

- Extra-virgin olive oil is a key ingredient in the Mediterranean diet. It's known as an anti-inflammatory oil due to a special component oleocanthal, which can halt the production of pro-inflammatory enzymes. You can reduce pain and inflammation by including olive oil in your diet. It has a smoke point of about 375 degrees.

- Grapeseed oil is suitable for high-heat cooking as well, with a smoke point of 420 degrees.

- Red palm oil is a good source of antioxidants and also offers anti-inflammatory components. It is suitable for high-heat cooking with a smoke point of 455 degrees.

- Rice bran oil is suitable for high-temperature cooking such as wok stir-fry and has a smoke point of 490 degrees.

- Walnut oil has a low smoke point of just 320 degrees, making it suitable for light sautéing. It's considered anti-inflammatory and is rich in omega-3 fatty acids.

Sweeteners

I recommend only a few natural sweeteners: stevia (SweetLeaf's Vanilla Crème stevia is very good), coconut sugar, coconut nectar, and xylitol made from organic birch bark (but not what is the by-product of the wood pulp industry). The only reliable brand I know is The Ultimate Sweetener made from 100 percent birch bark; you can order it online. Local raw honey or pure maple syrup may be used in limited amounts.

Whole grains

I recommend using only ancient grains, including brown rice, quinoa, millet, spelt (does have some gluten), amaranth, and kamut.

Animal protein (fish, chicken, turkey, and red meat)

Eat only clean meat and poultry, meaning no antibiotics or hormones and preferably animals that were raised cage-free, organic, and grass fed. Organic muscle meat has been shown to be much higher in conjugated linoleic acid (CLA) and omega-3 fatty acids than conventionally raised animals. And studies show that beef that is grass fed is four times higher in vitamin E than feedlot cattle.

When it comes to fish, buy only wild caught, including salmon and trout. Farm-raised fish are not a healthy choice. By buying wild-caught fish, you'll be able to avoid fish given antibiotics and hormones and raised in unhealthy conditions. For saltwater fish and seafood, it is best to stick to wild-caught Alaskan fish and seafood. Testing done by the Alaska Department of

Environmental Conservation has shown that radiation from the 2011 tsunami and subsequent nuclear disaster has not affected Alaskan fish or seafood.[2] Furthermore, most Atlantic salmon is farm-raised, which is not a healthy choice.

Legumes

Choosing organic beans, lentils, and split peas is best, and buy them locally grown if you can find them. I do not recommend eating soy foods except for a small amount of organic fermented soy products. Soy products are high in phytates, which inhibit the absorption of some minerals, including zinc, iron, and magnesium. Fermented soy products, however, have lower phytate content, so they are better for you than other soy products.[3] Organic is recommended because soy is the biggest GMO crop in the United States.

Plant milks

Choose plant milks from the following list:

- Coconut milk: Choose unsweetened coconut milk in cartons. Watch out for BPA-lined cans.

- Almond milk: Choose unsweetened milk that uses non-GMO almonds.

- Rice milk: Choose unsweetened milk, but be aware that rice milk is naturally higher in sugar than the other options.

It is processed milled rice blended with water; the carbohydrates in the rice become sugar.

- Hemp milk: Choose unsweetened milk. Hemp milk has more protein than other choices, with the exception of soy milk, which I don't recommend. Hemp milk is thick and creamy and has a strong taste, but it is good for soup.

Shopping Tip

Try to refrain from purchasing canned foods, but when you do, make it a habit to read the labels because many canned foods contain BPA. However, a number of companies have changed their cans to make them BPA-free due to consumer backlash. This is a great example of how our choices can change the market for the better.

WHY YOU SHOULD BUY ORGANIC FOOD

There are at least four good reasons to purchase organic food. First off, you're helping to reduce your body's overall toxic load. Organic produce has not been sprayed with pesticides, herbicides, or fungicides or been exposed to ionizing radiation. Organic meat comes from animals that have not been injected with hormones and antibiotics. Conventionally raised animals are mostly fed soy and corn, 90 percent of which is genetically modified. Conventionally raised dairy cows may be given genetically engineered rBGH hormone to increase milk production. This causes infections, so they are given large doses of antibiotics.

Have you ever wondered how eating organic might impact your health or that of your family? A 2005 study showed that in just fifteen days, children eating an organic diet experienced a dramatic decrease in organophosphorus pesticides.[4]

Choose organic to avoid GMOs, which are foods with changes made to their DNA in an abnormal way not found in nature. GMO foods do not come without health consequences, and these will be discussed further later in the chapter.

Organic farming is also good for our environment, especially since agriculture is one of the major factors affecting water pollution today.[5]

And perhaps the most important point of all is that organic produce has been shown to be more nutritious than conventionally grown food. For example, a "large meta-analysis published in 2014 in the *British Journal of Nutrition*, found that organic crops—ranging from carrots and broccoli to apples and blueberries—have substantially higher concentrations of a range of antioxidants and other potentially beneficial compounds."[6]

THE DIRTY DOZEN AND
THE CLEAN FIFTEEN

If you're working with a limited budget and can't afford to purchase only organic produce, at least avoid what the Environmental Working Group (EWG) calls "The Dirty Dozen." The EWG prepares a report each year on the top most heavily sprayed produce. You can even get an app for your phone to use when you shop to make sure you steer clear of the most contaminated fruits and vegetables. By just avoiding these top twelve, it is estimated that you can reduce your pesticide exposure by 90 percent.[7] The Dirty Dozen list changes each year. To get the current ratings, go to www.ewg.org.

The Dirty Dozen
Here is the Dirty Dozen List[8] as of 2017:

- Strawberries
- Spinach
- Nectarines
- Apples
- Peaches
- Pears
- Cherries
- Grapes
- Celery
- Tomatoes
- Sweet bell peppers
- Potatoes

The Clean Fifteen
The produce EWG lists in the Clean Fifteen have the least amount of pesticide spray residues, meaning these

foods are the safest to consume as conventional produce. As of 2017 the list includes:[9]

- Sweet corn
- Avocados
- Pineapples
- Cabbage
- Onions
- Sweet peas (frozen)
- Papayas
- Asparagus

- Mangos
- Eggplant
- Honeydew melon
- Kiwi
- Cantaloupe
- Cauliflower
- Grapefruit

WHAT ABOUT
MEXICAN ORGANICS?

Have you ever wondered whether you should opt for organic produce from Mexico or just go with the conventional option? In winter and early spring most of us don't have any local options. But that Mexican sticker can shoot up a red flag for some of us. How can we know that Mexican organics are reliable and safe for us to eat? As demand for organic produce in the United States has grown, Mexico's organic farmland has grown by 32 percent per year due to the increased demand.[10]

With a little digging, it seems that Mexican organics is a good option after all. Organics from Mexico must also meet the requirements of the USDA National Organics Program (NOP) standards, and they must be certified by a USDA-accredited agency. Certification goes beyond what many may think; it includes processing plants and farm field inspection. Farmers must provide detailed records. This means it must be grown without synthetic pesticides, sewage sludge, artificial fertilizers, genetically modified organisms (GMO), and irradiation. Mexico has organic certification agencies and the USDA has border inspections to ensure food safety. The United States has enforced the NOP since 2002, and the Mexican government has been enforcing its own regulations about organic products since 2006.[11]

It is estimated that Mexico has more than 110,000 organic farmers, and the vast majority (more than 90 percent) have fewer than nine acres on which to farm.[12] To support organic Mexican farmers is part of compassionate eating. Many small organic farmers take great pride in producing their food. This industry allows them to earn a wage and remain on their land and be part of their community rather than needing to relocate to a larger city where they can find work.

SHOULD YOU EAT IRRADIATED FOOD?

We seem so far removed from irradiated food because most of us have never seen it done, but it happens every day. Food is said to be irradiated to make it better for us, to destroy microorganisms, bacteria, viruses, or insects that might be in the food. However, it is important to avoid irradiated fruits and vegetables as much as you can.

A number of food producers rely on gamma radiation to kill pests, bacteria, and germs and to increase shelf life, but we lose nutrition because irradiation destroys vitamins, enzymes, phytonutrients, and biophotons. It also produces harmful free radicals that damage cells along with harmful radiolytic by-products known as thalidomides.[13]

Dr. George Tritsch of Roswell Park Memorial Institute, New York State Department of Health, says he is "opposed to consuming irradiated food because of the abundant and convincing evidence in the referenced scientific literature, that the condensation products of the free radicals formed during irradiation produce statistically significant increases in carcinogenesis, mutagenesis and cardiovascular disease in animals and man."[14]

Irradiating fruits and vegetables causes even greater problems than irradiating other foods because they have a larger water content, which allows more free radicals to form. Conquering food-borne illnesses will not be accomplished with irradiation. Instead, we must cease from overusing pesticides, which creates weak plants. And our overcrowded factory farms lead to sick animals. We need more humane farms and sanitary conditions in our plants that process foods.

AVOID GMO FOODS

It is estimated that up to 80 percent of our processed foods contain genetically modified organisms (GMO), which means they are bioengineered.[15] Despite many people's acceptance of GMO foods, there are dangers that we should be aware of before consuming such food. In fact, there are many reasons you should avoid GMO foods entirely.

GMO foods should be avoided because they are unhealthy for humans. GMO foods can cause organ damage, affect the gastrointestinal tract and the immune system, cause infertility, and even accelerate the aging process.[16] For example, GMO corn was combined with a bacteria to produce its own insecticide, Bt toxin, which kills insects by destroying the lining of their intestinal tracts. But it isn't just insects that it harms. It can also poke holes in human intestinal tracts, causing intestinal and digestive issues. And this toxin can't be washed off. It becomes part of the matrix of the plant.[17]

Monsanto researchers studied three strains of GM maize (corn) fed to animals, and the animals showed signs of liver and kidney damage. Of these strains, two of them were genetically modified to synthesize insecticide toxins, and the third was manipulated to resist herbicides.[18] These three strains of GMO corn are grown for humans to eat in America. Reports show that Monsanto released this information only after a legal challenge from Greenpeace and other groups against GMO foods.[19]

In the Monsanto study unusual levels of hormones were found in the blood and urine of rats that were fed the maize for three months when compared to rats that were fed a non-GM diet. And higher levels of blood sugar and triglycerides were found in the female rats, and higher blood sugar and triglyceride levels can contribute to weight gain, insulin resistance, and metabolic syndrome. The researchers concluded, "Effects were mostly associated with the kidney and liver, the dietary detoxifying organs, although different between the 3 GMOs. Other effects were also noticed in the heart, adrenal glands, [and] spleen."[20]

Another reason to stay away from GMO foods, according to Jeffrey Smith, founder of the Institute for Responsible Technology, is that GMO foods actually increase herbicide use by engineering crops that are more tolerant of them. "Between 1996 and 2008, US farmers sprayed an extra 383 million pounds of herbicide on GMOs."[21] This overabundance of herbicides, including Roundup, has since resulted in weeds that are also resistant to the herbicide, which in turn causes farmers to use even more of the herbicide. It is a downward spiral. "Not only does this create environmental harm, GM foods contain higher residues of toxic herbicides. Roundup, for example, is linked with sterility, hormone disruption, birth defects, and cancer."[22]

Soybeans and corn are the most widely grown GMO crops worldwide, followed by beets and alfalfa. But some potatoes, papaya, squash, tomato, flax, and more are also GMOs. According to Deborah Whitman, "Globally, acreage of GM crops has increased 25-fold in just 5 years, from approximately 4.3 million acres in 1996 to 109 million acres in 2000....Approximately 99 million acres were devoted to GM crops in the U.S. and Argentina alone."[23]

Genetically modified foods are everywhere—from grocery store shelves to restaurants to vending machines. And worse, there is no labeling required. We may never know we're eating GMOs. Just recently I had a test that indicated I'd eaten some GMO food. I'm one of the strictest people I know with regards to my diet, and I have no idea where I got GMO food from. Without mandatory labeling, we may never know for certain whether or not we are eating GMO food. This is one reason some health practitioners believe food allergies are on the rise. You might get a vegetable of some sort spliced with a peanut or other nut gene and have a reaction without ever knowing why.

You can avoid GMO foods by becoming a smart shopper. Be aware of the top genetically engineered crops. Some experts estimate that up to thirty thousand different products on grocery store shelves are genetically modified; that number is so high because a good percentage of foods contain soy. About 90 percent of our soy crop in America is GMO.[24]

To obtain a GMO shopping guide, go to www.non gmoshoppingguide.com.

CHAPTER 8

SOUP RECIPES TO CLEANSE YOUR BODY, ENCOURAGE WEIGHT LOSS, RESTORE HEALTH, AND INCREASE ENERGY

A good broth can raise the dead.

—SOUTH AMERICAN PROVERB

SOUP IS A great way to cleanse your body, lose weight, restore your health, and increase energy. It's also a great way to use leftovers.

This chapter contains plenty of recipes to get you started in souping. As you begin, remember that most soup recipes are easily adaptable to your personal preference. If a soup has something you don't like, omit it. If it's missing something you know you'd love, go ahead and add it. And don't let the time it takes to cook deter you; a soup may need to simmer for a while, but it doesn't require you to stand there while it cooks. You can relax or do chores around the house while it simmers. But if you are really pressed for time, you can prepare a simple blender soup in just a few minutes. Many quick-to-make soups are still healthy and yummy. You can also use premade broth and frozen vegetables as time savers.

Also, as mentioned previously, soup is great to refrigerate or freeze for later. You can make plenty when you have time to have on hand for days when you don't have time to cook, don't feel like cooking, or are a bit under the weather.

RAW BLENDER SOUPS

In the summer we are presented with bountiful produce. Soup is a perfect way to use this produce. Chilled soups are great for warm summer days. You can blend fresh, colorful produce that is sun-ripened and rich in nutrients. These soups are a refreshing way start any meal or to start your day, or they might be the meal itself. Blended soups pair well with lighter meals such as salads and wraps. For many more blended raw soup (smoothie) recipes, get my book *The Juice Lady's Big Book of Juices and Green Smoothies*. It has more than four hundred great recipes.

CARIBBEAN MORNING

1 cup coconut milk
½ cup fresh orange juice (about ½ large orange, juiced)
1 Tbsp. coconut oil
1 cup papaya chunks, fresh or frozen

1 cup pineapple chunks, fresh or frozen

½ cup kale, chopped

2 Tbsp. unsweetened coconut, shredded

6 ice cubes (optional; not needed if using frozen fruit)

Pour the coconut milk, orange juice, and coconut oil in a blender and blend until combined. Then add papaya, pineapple, kale, shredded coconut, and ice cubes; blend again until smooth. Serves 2.

CREAMY CUCUMBER SOUP

This is a filling, satisfying cold soup.

1½ cups fresh cucumber juice (2 cucumbers, juiced)

¼ cup fresh lemon juice (about 2 lemons, juiced)

1 Tbsp. green onions, chopped

1 Tbsp. red onion, chopped

1 Tbsp. fresh parsley, chopped

1 large ripe avocado, peeled and seeded

1 garlic clove, minced

1 tsp. tamari or coconut aminos

1–2 tsp. curry powder, or to taste

½ tsp. ground cumin

1 Tbsp. fresh basil, chopped

Blend all ingredients except basil until smooth. To make the soup thinner, if necessary, add a little more cucumber or lemon juice. Ladle soup into bowls and garnish with fresh basil. Serve cold. Serves 2.

ENERGY BOOST

½ cup fresh carrot juice (3–4 medium carrots, juiced)
½ cup fresh apple juice (about 1½ apples, juiced)
1 Tbsp. fresh lemon juice (about ½ lemon)
½ cup packed baby spinach
½ cup raw cashews
6 ice cubes

Place all ingredients in a blender and blend until creamy and smooth. Serves 1.

MINTY GREEN DELIGHT

1 avocado, peeled, seeded, and cut in quarters
1 cup raw spinach
½ English cucumber, peeled and cut in chunks
½–¾ cup coconut milk
2 Tbsp. fresh lime juice (1 lime, juiced)
1 Tbsp. green powder of choice (optional)
2–3 Tbsp. ground almonds (optional)

Combine all ingredients except almonds in a blender and blend until smooth. Sprinkle ground almonds on top, as desired. Serves 2.

REFRESHING CARROT GINGER SOUP

This recipe is one of the favorites that my husband and I serve at our juice and raw-foods retreat.

> 3 cups carrot juice (15–21 carrots, juiced, depending on size)
> 1 avocado, peeled and seeded
> ¼ cup fresh lime juice (2–3 limes, juiced)
> 1 Tbsp. minced ginger
> ¼ tsp. sea salt
> ¼ small shallot

Pour everything in a blender and process until well combined. Serves 2–3.

REFRESHING TOMATO BASIL SOUP

> 3 medium tomatoes
> ¼ cucumber, peeled
> 2 Tbsp. fresh lemon juice (1 lemon, juiced)
> 1 avocado, peeled and seeded
> 2 Tbsp. fresh basil, chopped
> 1 small garlic clove
> Fresh basil leaves for garnish, chopped (optional)

In a blender blend the tomatoes until chunky. Add the cucumber, lemon, avocado, basil, and garlic. Blend well. Pour into bowls and garnish with fresh basil leaves, as desired. Serves 2.

SOUTHWEST ENERGY SOUP

This is fast soup for a busy day.

1 cup fresh carrot juice (5–7 medium carrots, juiced)
2 Tbsp. lemon juice (1 lemon, peeled if not organic, juiced)
1 tsp. ginger juice (1-inch-chunk ginger root, juiced)
1 avocado, peeled and seeded
½ tsp. ground cumin

Pour the juices in a blender. Add the avocado and cumin and blend until smooth. Serve chilled. Serves 1.

SWEET WATERCRESS SOUP

1 cup coconut milk (or other unsweetened plant milk)
1 cup chopped watercress
1–2 cups fresh or frozen berries
6 ice cubes (optional, may not be needed if using frozen fruit)
Several drops of liquid stevia (optional)

Combine all ingredients in a blender and process well until smooth and creamy/slushy. Serve as soon as possible. Serves 1.

YUMMY GREEN SOUP

1 Tbsp. lime juice (½ lime, juiced)
1 tsp. ginger juice (1-inch-chunk ginger, juiced)
1 avocado, peeled, seeded, and cut in quarters

1 cup raw spinach
½ English cucumber, peeled and cut in chunks
1 Tbsp. green powder of choice (optional)
2–3 Tbsp. ground almonds (optional)

Pour the lime and ginger juice into a blender with the avocado, spinach, cucumber, and green powder. Blend until smooth. Sprinkle ground almonds on top, as desired. Serves 2.

YUMMY YAM BISQUE

This soup tastes similar to pumpkin pie.

1½ cups yam juice (about 2 large yams, juiced)
1 cup almond, oat, or rice milk
¼ cup red onion, chopped
1 avocado, peeled and seeded
1 tsp. nutmeg
¼ tsp. cinnamon
¼ tsp. ground allspice
¼ tsp. ground mace
¼ tsp. cardamom

After juicing the yams to yield about 1½ cup of juice, let the juice sit in a large measuring cup or bowl until the starch settles to the bottom. It will look thick and white. This should take about an hour. Pour the clear juice at the top into the blender, but leave out the starch because it will make the soup gritty. Add the milk, onion, and avocado and blend until smooth. Add the spices and blend until smooth. Serves 2.

ZIPPY GAZPACHO

This is a low-carb gluten-free version of classic gazpacho.

3 pounds tomatoes, peeled, seeded, and chopped
1 cucumber, peeled and chopped
1 cup celery, chopped
1 Tbsp. red bell pepper, chopped
½ cup red onion, chopped
1 tsp. garlic, chopped
1 Tbsp. jalapeño pepper, chopped
3 Tbsp. red wine vinegar
¼ cup extra-virgin olive oil
1½ cups tomato juice
Sea salt, to taste
Freshly ground black pepper, to taste
Pinch of ground coriander
¼ cup cilantro, chopped
1 Tbsp. lime juice (½ lime, juiced)

Topping

2 Tbsp. red bell pepper, diced
2 Tbsp. cucumber, diced
2 Tbsp. red onion, diced
2 Tbsp. tomatoes, diced
2 Tbsp. cilantro, chopped
1 tsp. minced garlic

1 tsp. fresh lime juice (⅓ lime, juiced)

1 tsp. extra-virgin olive oil

Sea salt, to taste

Freshly ground black pepper, to taste

Put all ingredients except for topping ingredients into blender and blend until smooth. Pour mixture into a bowl and chill for 4 hours. While the soup is being chilled, combine all topping ingredients. After 4 hours, ladle the soup into bowls and top with a large spoonful of the topping. Serves 8.

GENTLY WARMED SOUPS

BROCCOLI SOUP

1 cup vegetable stock

1–2 cups broccoli, chopped

½ onion, chopped

1 red or yellow bell pepper, chopped

1–2 stalks celery, chopped

1 avocado, peeled and seeded

1 tsp. Celtic sea salt

½ tsp. cumin

1 tsp. grated ginger (optional)

Squeeze of lemon (optional)

Gently warm the vegetable stock, keeping the temperature at 115 degrees or below. Add the broccoli and onion and warm for 5 minutes. Turn off the heat. Then add the bell pepper and celery and leave it for an additional

5 minutes. Pour the mixture into a blender and puree it until smooth. Add the avocado and blend until smooth. Add the sea salt and cumin and then blend. Pour soup into bowls. If using ginger, add to the top of the soup and stir in. A squeeze of lemon is nice, as well; add as desired. Serves 2.

CREAM OF CAULIFLOWER SOUP

½ onion, chopped
3 stalks celery, chopped
1 head cauliflower, chopped
1 Tbsp. virgin coconut oil
1 cup almond or rice milk
½ tsp. sea salt
Pepper to taste (optional)

Lightly steam onion, celery, and cauliflower for about 5 minutes or until just tender. Combine in a blender with the coconut oil, milk, and salt. Blend well. Pour into bowls. Serves 2.

RED VELVET SOUP

3 large red bell peppers, cut into chunks
4 garlic cloves
1 cup unsweetened almond, oat, or coconut milk
1 Tbsp. balsamic vinegar
2 tsp. sea salt
¼ cup fresh basil
2 Tbsp. fresh basil, chopped, for garnish

Lightly steam the peppers and garlic for about 5 minutes or just until tender. Pour the milk into a blender and add the peppers, garlic, balsamic vinegar, salt, and ¼ cup basil. Blend on high speed until smooth. Pour into bowls and garnish with fresh basil as desired. Serve immediately. Serves 1–2.

CREAMY SOUPS
(WITHOUT THE CREAM)

It's easy to make a creamy soup without any dairy products. You can use cashews, rice, almond butter, cashew butter, or a plant milk such as almond, coconut, or hemp. You can add some arrowroot to thicken these soups, and you can blend part or all of the soup until it is creamy.

CREAMY CURRIED CARROT SOUP

Cashews or rice will thicken the soup and make it creamier.

    2 Tbsp. extra-virgin olive oil
    1 yellow onion, chopped
    1 tsp. sea salt
    2 lb. carrots, cut into ½-inch pieces
    2 garlic cloves, minced
    5 cups vegetable stock
    ½ cup cooked brown rice or raw cashews, soaked 30
        minutes and drained
    2-inch-chunk ginger, peeled and chopped
    1 Tbsp. curry powder

1 Tbsp. fresh lemon juice (½ lemon, juiced)

Sea salt, to taste

Freshly ground black pepper, to taste

Add the olive oil to a large stock pot and heat over medium heat. Once the oil is heated, add the onion and salt, and sauté for 5 minutes. Then add the carrots and garlic, cover, and cook for 5 more minutes. After cooking the carrots, add the vegetable stock and the cooked rice or cashews. Bring the soup to a boil and reduce the heat. Allow it to simmer for 25 minutes. Separate the soup into batches and puree; make sure not to fill the blender too much!

As you puree, add the ginger and curry powder into the soup. After the soup is pureed, stir in the lemon juice and season with salt and pepper to taste. Serves 6–8.

CREAMY SPRING ASPARAGUS SOUP

¼ cup extra-virgin olive oil

2 garlic cloves, chopped

½ cup onion, diced

5 cups fresh asparagus, cut into 1-inch pieces
    (2 bunches)

4 cups vegetable stock, to cover

¼ bunch parsley, roughly chopped

1½ tsp. sea salt (or more to taste)

Freshly ground black pepper, to taste

1–2 cups coconut milk, or to taste

1 Tbsp. fresh lemon juice (½ lemon, juiced)

Fresh purified water, as needed

Chopped parsley for garnish to taste (optional)

Vegan yogurt or vegan sour cream to taste (optional)

In a large soup pot add the oil and heat over medium heat. Stir in the garlic and onion. Add the asparagus and just enough stock to cover the vegetables—but no more. You can add more later to thin the soup if necessary.

Add the chopped parsley and season to taste with sea salt and fresh pepper. Bring the soup to a high simmer before covering the soup and reducing the heat to medium heat. Let it simmer for about 20 minute or until the asparagus are fork tender. Then remove the soup from the heat and use an immersion blender (or divide in batches and pour in your blender) to puree the soup. Once the soup is pureed, return it to the heat and add the coconut milk and lemon juice. Stir and heat through gently (don't boil the pureed soup). Taste test and adjust seasonings.

Garnish with fresh minced parsley or a spoonful of plain vegan yogurt or vegan sour cream. Serves 6.

SWEET HARVEST CREAM OF CARROT

This soup was created by my friend Chef Jeff for this book. It uses full-fat coconut milk for its creamy consistency.

2 lb. carrots, scrubbed and cut into 1-inch pieces

1 large onion, medium diced

½ tsp. cinnamon

¼ tsp. cloves

¼ tsp. allspice

¼ tsp. nutmeg

10 cups purified water

1 cup full-fat coconut milk

1 tsp. sea salt or to taste

½ tsp. freshly ground black pepper or to taste

Place large soup pot over medium heat and add all ingredients except for the coconut milk, salt, and pepper. Cook for one hour until carrots are fork tender. Puree until smooth and creamy. Add coconut milk and continue to puree. Season with salt and pepper to desired taste. Serves 6–8.

What Is Purified Water?

Purified water has had chemicals and contaminants removed from it. There are many types of purified water: bottled spring water, distilled, reverse osmosis, carbon filtration, and deionization. We all know how important drinking purified water is; similarly, you don't want to pour contaminated water into your soup pot.

CREAMY TOMATO BASIL SOUP

This creamy tomato soup recipe is delicious and was created by my friend Chef Jeff for this book. It utilizes coconut milk and pureed veggies to make the creamy consistency.

2 Tbsp. extra-virgin olive oil

1 large onion, small diced

6 garlic cloves, minced

½ tsp. chili flakes

4 roma tomatoes, small diced

2 28-oz. cans crushed tomatoes

2 cups vegetable broth

1 cup coconut milk

1 tsp. sea salt

½ Tbsp. pepper

¼ cup chopped fresh basil

½ cup parsley, chopped (for garnish)

Put olive oil in a large pot over medium heat and add onion, garlic, and chili flakes; cook until translucent, about 5 minutes. Add the diced tomatoes, stir to combine and cook for an additional 5 minutes.

Add the cans of crushed tomatoes and vegetable broth. Simmer for one hour; stir about every 10 minutes to avoid scorching on the bottom.

Add the coconut milk, salt, pepper, and basil. Simmer for a few minutes while stirring to make sure all ingredients are well incorporated. Garnish with chopped parsley. Serves 6–8.

CURRIED CREAMY GREEN PEA SOUP

Fresh green peas give this bright green soup a very different flavor from dried split peas. This soup is a great accompaniment to a Middle Eastern dish, and it is nice served with hummus or baba ganoush.

1 Tbsp. extra-virgin olive oil
1 medium yellow onion, chopped
1 medium red onion, chopped
4 garlic cloves, minced
½ cup cilantro, chopped
3 Tbsp. curry powder
Sea salt to taste
Freshly ground pepper, to taste
3½ cup fresh shelled peas
2 16-ounce packages frozen peas, thawed and drained
3-4 cups vegetable or chicken stock
Cilantro, chopped, for garnish (optional)
Toasted sunflower seeds (optional)
Unsweetened vegan yogurt (optional)

In a large soup pot over medium heat, add the oil and then sauté onions and garlic until translucent (about 5 minutes). Add the cilantro, curry, salt, and pepper. Cook over medium heat, stirring occasionally, for about 15 minutes. Add the peas and cook for 5 minutes. Add the stock and simmer for another 10 minutes. Let cool a bit. Divide into parts and puree until smooth and creamy.

Ladle the soup into bowls and garnish with chopped cilantro and toasted sunflower seeds or a dollop of unsweetened vegan yogurt. Serves 4.

VEGETABLE SOUPS

How to Make a Vegetable Stock

Add vegetables such as onion, garlic, celery, and carrots to a stockpot. Sauté for about 5 minutes. Fill the pot with water and add vegetable scraps and frozen vegetables along with herbs of choice. Let it simmer for 45 minutes. Strain and you have vegetable stock.

COCONUT CORN CHOWDER

This is an original recipe by Chef Jeff created for this book.

2 Tbsp. extra-virgin olive oil
1 large onion, small diced
5 celery stalks, small diced
4 large carrots, small diced
4 garlic cloves, minced
5 cups vegetable broth
2 14-ounce cans unsweetened coconut milk
6 small gold potatoes, small diced
3 lb. corn kernels, fresh or frozen
¼ cup chives
¼ cup parsley
3 Tbsp. arrowroot in 6 Tbsp. cold water (mixed together until smooth)
1 tsp. sea salt
½ Tbsp. pepper

Put olive oil in a large pot over medium heat and add onion, celery, carrots, and garlic; cook until translucent, about 5 minutes. Then add vegetable broth and coconut milk and bring to a boil. Reduce heat, add the potatoes and simmer for approximately 30 minutes or until potatoes are soft. Then add the corn, chives, parsley, arrowroot, salt, and pepper. Cook for another 10 minutes or until desired thickness and serve. Serves 8.

CREAMY THREE-MUSHROOM SOUP

½ lb. fresh button mushrooms
¼ lb. fresh oyster mushrooms or 1 ounce, dried
¼ lb. fresh shiitake mushrooms or 1 ounce, dried
2–4 Tbsp. virgin coconut oil or extra-virgin olive oil
2 whole shallots, minced
3 cups unsweetened coconut milk
Sea salt to taste
Ground black pepper to taste
4 egg yolks

First prepare the fresh mushrooms by cleaning them and removing the caps from the stems. If you prefer, you can separate the fresh mushroom caps into two groups and slice half into ⅛-inch slices and add the other caps with the stems and dried mushrooms. (Otherwise, combine all caps and stems and chop them finely.

If using dried mushrooms, soak them in hot water for 20–30 minutes. Then drain the water and squeeze out the excess and chop them finely. Place them with the fresh mushroom stems (or stems and caps if you aren't using sliced caps).

Next, prepare the shallots by peeling and mincing them.

If you chose to slice the mushroom caps, then heat 1 tablespoon of oil in a stainless steel skillet over medium-high heat. When the oil is warm, add the sliced caps to the skillet. Sauté for about 5 minutes or until the caps just begin to change color. Then remove them from the skillet and set to the side. Then add the remaining oil to the skillet; when everything is warm, add the remaining mushrooms and the shallots to the skillet and sauté for about 10 minutes (they should be tender). If not using sliced mushroom caps, heat the oil in a stainless steel skillet. When the oil is warm, add the mushrooms and shallots to the skillet and cook until they are tender, about 10 minutes.

Next place the chopped mushrooms (not the slices, if used), shallots, and milk in a medium saucepan, and heat over medium-low heat. Then season the soup with salt and pepper to taste and then continue to simmer for another 20–25 minutes.

Meanwhile, place egg yolks in a bowl and whisk until they are light and lemon colored. Then, once the soup has simmered for the recommended amount of time, whisk ½ cup of the soup mixture into eggs. Do this only 2 tablespoons at a time.

Next beat the egg mixture into the rest of the soup by pouring in a slow and steady stream and beating as you go. Add sliced mushroom caps, if used, and heat the soup thoroughly, but do not bring it to a boil. Serves 4.

FAT-BURNING CABBAGE SOUP

1 Tbsp. extra-virgin olive oil

4 garlic cloves, minced

1 large yellow onion, diced

½ lb. carrots, scrubbed and sliced

1 cup celery, chopped

½ cup zucchini, chopped

½ lb. frozen green beans

1 28-oz. can diced tomatoes

1 8-oz. can tomato sauce or tomato juice

1 head green cabbage, chopped in 1-inch pieces

6 cups vegetable or beef broth

½ cup fresh parsley, chopped

½ Tbsp. smoked paprika

1 tsp. dried oregano

½ tsp. dried thyme

Freshly ground black pepper to taste

Sea salt to taste

1–2 Tbsp. fresh lemon juice (about 1 small lemon, juiced)

Add olive oil, garlic, and onion to a large stockpot and sauté over medium heat until the onions are soft and transparent. Then add the carrots, celery, zucchini, green beans, diced tomatoes (with juice), and tomato sauce or juice to the pot. Stir to combine.

Let the vegetables heat, and then add the cabbage. Add the broth, parsley, paprika, oregano, thyme, and pepper, and then stir.

Cover the pot and bring it to a boil. Once boiling, reduce heat to medium-low and allow the soup to simmer for about 20 minutes, or until the cabbage is tender and soft. Remove the soup from heat and add salt to taste, starting with small amounts at first. Stir in lemon juice. Serves 12–15.

RUSSIAN VEGETARIAN BORSCH

This recipe was created by Chef Jeff for this book.

8 cups water
1 tsp. sea salt
3 medium beets
3 medium potatoes, cut into small pieces
½ head cabbage, thinly shredded
2 Tbsp. olive oil
2 carrots, grated
1 medium onion, medium diced
4 garlic cloves, minced
3 Tbsp. tomato paste
8 cups vegetable broth
4 Tbsp. lemon juice
¼ tsp. freshly ground pepper
2 bay leaves
¼ cup fresh parsley, chopped

1 Tbsp. fresh or dry dill

Fresh parsley, chopped (for garnish)

In a large stockpot pour in water and salt. Add washed beets; cover and boil for about an hour. Once you can easily pierce the beets with a fork, remove them from the water and set aside to cool, keeping the water.

Add the potatoes to the water and boil 15–20 minutes. Add the thinly shredded cabbage when the potatoes are halfway done.

Pour the olive oil into a sauté pan on medium-high heat, add carrots, onion, and garlic and sauté for 8 minutes or until soft, then stir in tomato paste and add all of it to the pot. Finely chop the beets and add them to the pot. Add vegetable broth, lemon juice, pepper, bay leaves, parsley, and dill in the pot. Simmer for an additional 10 minutes; remove the bay leaves. Serve soup garnished with chopped parsley. Serves 8–10.

HEALING SOUPS

BONE BROTH

4–5 grass-fed beef bones, chicken bones, or any mixture of bones from wild or pasture-raised, healthy animals (if using beef bones, I prefer meaty beef shank)

Purified water

1 Tbsp. raw apple cider vinegar

1 carrot, chopped

¼ onion

1 clove garlic

Sea salt and pepper

Place bones into a large soup pot or crockpot. Fill your pot with filtered water to cover the bones. Add the vinegar, carrot, onion, and garlic.

Turn your heat on low for the soup pot or set your Crock-Pot on low. Simmer for 24 hours. (I put my soup pot in the oven on 200 degrees overnight.) Poultry bones can simmer as long as 24 hours, and beef bones can simmer for up to 48 hours.

Use tongs to remove the bones, and then pour the broth through a sieve into storage containers. Season with salt and pepper to taste. Store in the refrigerator. It should keep for 5–7 days, or you can freeze it for later. Skim fat layer off the top, if it forms.

HEALING GREEN MUNG BEAN SOUP[1]

Mung beans act as an anti-inflammatory. In Ayurveda medicine mung bean soup is known to help balance the body. Its spices and penetrating herbs are the driving force to help rid the body of toxins and mucus that lodges there over time due to poor diet, lack of exercise, and an unhealthy lifestyle. This soup helps to break down mucus and flush it out of the body.

1 cup whole green mung beans

2 cups purified water plus ½ tsp. sea salt (to cook beans)

1 Tbsp. coconut oil or extra-virgin olive oil

½ tsp. mustard seeds

¼ tsp. hing (Eastern spice, optional)

1 bay leaf

½ tsp. turmeric

½ tsp. cumin

1–2 tsp. coriander powder

2 tsp. ginger, finely chopped

1 tsp. garlic, finely chopped

½ onion chopped

1 carrot, chopped

1 rib celery, chopped

Freshly ground black pepper, to taste

2 cups purified water (for the soup)

1 tsp. sea salt

2 tsp. fresh lemon juice

Soak the mung beans for several hours or overnight in purified water. Then drain the beans and wash them twice. Cook the beans either in a pressure cooker or soup pot with 2 cups water and salt until tender. The pressure cooker will be faster, taking around 25 minutes until the beans are done completely. The beans must be tender and cooked completely.

Heat the oil in a large stockpot and add the mustard seeds. When the mustard seeds begin to pop, add the hing (if using), bay leaf, turmeric, cumin, coriander, ginger, garlic, onion, carrot, celery, and a pinch of black pepper. Mix well and sauté until the vegetables are tender. Make sure the soup does not burn.

Add the cooked beans, water, and salt to the soup pot.

Bring the soup to a boil and simmer for 15 minutes. Add the lemon juice, remove the bay leaf, and serve. Serves 6.

LEMON GARLIC SOUP

The garlic makes this a very healing soup.

    1 Tbsp. extra-virgin olive oil
    1 Tbsp. fresh garlic, minced
    6 cups chicken or vegetable broth
    2 eggs
    ⅓–½ cup fresh lemon juice (2–3 lemons, juiced)
    1 Tbsp. arrowroot powder
    ¼ tsp. freshly ground black pepper
    ½ tsp. curcumin
    ¼ cup fresh cilantro or parsley, chopped (for garnish)

In a 4-quart stockpot heat the olive oil over medium-high heat and sauté the garlic for 1–2 minutes, or until just fragrant. Do not let the garlic brown.

Reserve ½ cup of the stock to mix with the eggs. Pour the remaining 5½ cups of stock into the pot with the garlic. Let the mixture come to a simmer.

In a small bowl whisk together the eggs, lemon juice, arrowroot, pepper, curcumin, and the ½ cup of reserved broth. Pour the mixture into the simmering stock and stir until it all thickens, which will take only a few minutes.

Serve the soup hot and garnish with fresh cilantro or parsley. Serves 4.

DETOX SOUPS

Turmeric helps detox the liver

Turmeric, a member of the ginger family, has been shown in studies to have anti-inflammatory effects. Your liver is one of the most important detoxifying organs of the body. And turmeric is one of the best detoxifiers of the liver. Curcumin is a phytonutrient that gives turmeric its bright yellow color. According to the University of Maryland Medical Center, curcumin can encourage bile production within the gallbladder. This bile is used within the liver to help remove toxins from the body as well as to rejuvenate the liver. Because of this, turmeric has been accepted by some as a treatment for digestion and liver disorders. You can easily add more turmeric to your diet in soups, juice, tea, and curry. This spice can help you detox and prevent diseases such as cancer.[2]

COLOR ME GREEN DETOX SOUP

5 garlic cloves, minced
1 Tbsp. extra-virgin olive oil
½ tsp. sea salt
1 cup broccoli, chopped
1–1½ cups spinach
1 cup kale, chopped
1 can cannellini or great northern beans, drained
2 tsp. fresh turmeric, chopped or 1 tsp. dried turmeric
¼ cup lemon juice (1½ lemons, juiced)
1 large bunch of cilantro, chopped

1 Tbsp. all-purpose seasoning
1 bouillon cube
3½ cups of water
Sea salt and pepper to taste

Combine garlic, olive oil, and salt in a large soup pot; turn on stove to medium heat and sauté until the mixture becomes aromatic, for about 1–2 minutes. Then add the chopped broccoli and stir for 5 more minutes.

Add the spinach and stir the mixture together until the spinach leaves are wilted. Add the kale, beans, turmeric, lemon juice, cilantro, all-purpose seasoning, bouillon, water, and salt and pepper to taste. Stir the mixture together and simmer for 15 minutes on low to medium heat. Remove the soup from the heat and blend everything together. Serves 2.

ITALIAN LENTIL DETOX SOUP

Created by Chef Jeff for this book, this soup has lots of garlic and vegetables to help your body remove toxins.

½ cup olive oil (divided, save some for garnish)
1 onion, medium diced
6 garlic cloves, minced
2 cups carrots, medium diced
2 cups butternut squash, medium diced
10 cups vegetable broth
2 cups green lentils
2 bay leaves
1 cup parsley, chopped (divided, save half for garnish)

2–3 cups kale, stem removed, chopped
1 tsp. sea salt, or to taste
Freshly ground pepper, to taste

Pour 2 tablespoons of olive oil into a large stockpot on medium heat. Add onion, garlic, carrots, and butternut squash, and sauté for 10 minutes. Add the vegetable broth, lentils, bay leaves, and parsley, and simmer for 1 hour or until the lentils are soft. Then stir in the kale and simmer for an additional 12 minutes until the kale is soft. Add salt and pepper to taste. When serving, add olive oil and parsley to each bowl to get a true Italian taste. Serves 6.

SPICY DETOX SOUP

1–2 Tbsp. extra-virgin olive oil
1 yellow onion, diced
1–2 Tbsp. fresh ginger, grated or finely minced
4–5 garlic cloves, grated or finely minced
1 medium zucchini, chopped
2 tsp. turmeric powder (or 3 tsp. fresh turmeric, finely grated)
¼ tsp. mustard seed (optional)
1 tsp. ground cumin
1 tsp. coriander
⅛ tsp. cayenne pepper, or to taste
4 cups purified water
4 cups veggie or chicken stock
1 tsp. sea salt

1–3 tsp. apple cider vinegar or lime or lemon juice (to taste)

½ cup brown rice (dry)

1 cup cooked garbanzo beans (or canned, drained)

1 can diced fire-roasted tomatoes (or use 1–2 cups fresh, diced tomatoes)

Cilantro, as garnish (optional)

In a large soup pot heat the oil over medium heat and add the onion. Sauté the onion for 2–3 minutes, and then add the ginger and lower the heat to medium low. Sauté for 5 minutes until the ginger begins to brown. Stir frequently. Add the garlic and zucchini and sauté for 2 more minutes. Then add all the spices and let heat for 1 more minute. Add the water, stock, and sea salt, and then bring the soup to a simmer. Then add the vinegar or citrus. (Feel free to adjust the salt, vinegar (or citrus), and spice level to your tastes.) Add the brown rice, beans, and tomatoes. Simmer for 30–40 minutes or until the rice is done. Serve and garnish with cilantro as desired. Serves 6.

You can refrigerate or freeze this soup in batches for later use.

WATERCRESS DETOX SOUP

This soup can also be used for weight loss as well as detox.

2 Tbsp. coconut oil

2 cups sweet onion, diced

1 cup celery, diced

1 tsp. sea salt to taste

4 medium zucchini, diced (yields about 8 cups)

4 cups vegetable, chicken, or bone broth

¼ cup unsweetened almond butter, creamy or crunchy

2 cups watercress, chopped

2 tsp. fresh lemon juice (⅓ lemon, juiced)

Freshly ground pepper to taste

¼ cup parsley, chopped

In a medium to large soup pot over medium heat, heat the oil and sauté the onion and celery with half the salt for about 5 minutes, or until translucent. Add the zucchini and sauté for 3 minutes.

Add the vegetable broth and the other ½ teaspoon salt. Stir in the almond butter until well combined. Increase the heat to high and bring to a boil. Reduce the heat to low and simmer for about 5 minutes or until the zucchini is tender. Add the watercress and let it simmer for about 5 minutes. Turn off the heat and cool the soup slightly. Stir in the lemon juice.

If you want a creamy soup, pour it into a blender in batches and puree until smooth and creamy. Return the soup to the soup pot, season to taste, and warm over low heat. Last stir in the parsley. Serves 4.

Note: I have blended this soup on low, so it's slightly chunky. I've also blended it on high, so it's very creamy. I can't decide which I like the most. You can add garlic, curry, or chopped scallions for variations.

SOUPS WITH LEGUMES

CHIPOTLE BEAN SOUP

1 Tbsp. virgin coconut oil
1 onion, chopped
1½ cups dried navy, lima, or pinto beans, soak beans overnight
1 clove garlic, chopped
2 chipotle chiles*, soaked 10 minutes in cold water
4 cups water or vegetable stock
2 tsp. Celtic sea salt
2 tsp. brown rice vinegar
Freshly ground pepper to taste

Heat oil in a large soup pot and cook onions over medium heat until soft. Drain the beans and add them to the onions along with garlic, chilies, and water or stock. Bring heat to high until mixture starts to boil. Reduce heat to low and cook for 1 hour or until the beans are soft. Remove chilies. For thicker, creamier soup, puree half the soup in a blender and then return it to the soup pot and mix well. Add the salt, vinegar, and pepper. Serves 4–6.

*Chipotle chilies add a smoked flavor that is similar to cooking beans with ham.

HERB AND VEGGIE SPLIT PEA SOUP

This thick, nourishing split pea soup with lots of vegetables and herbs is a filling soup, even for men.

    2 Tbsp. extra-virgin olive oil
    1 large onion, chopped
    3 large garlic cloves, minced
    2 cups split peas, washed and picked over
    2½ quarts purified water or vegetable stock
    1 Tbsp. vegetable base or 2 vegetable bouillon cubes
    1 small potato, peeled and chopped
    1 cup carrots, chopped
    1 cup celery, chopped
    ½ cup baby spinach
    ¼ cup parsley, chopped
    1 tsp. dried basil
    1 tsp. dried thyme
    1 tsp. dried marjoram
    1 tsp. dried oregano
    1 tsp. dried tarragon
    Sea salt to taste
    Freshly ground pepper to taste
    Unsweetened vegan yogurt, garnish

Put the oil in a large stock pot over medium heat. Add the onions and garlic and sauté for 5 minutes before adding split peas, water or vegetable stock, and vegetable base or bouillon. Heat the soup until it boils and then lower the heat, cover, and simmer for 1 hour.

Add the potato, carrots, celery, spinach, parsley, basil, thyme, marjoram, oregano, and tarragon. Simmer for 30 minutes. Stir in the salt and pepper to taste. For a smooth and creamy soup, divide it into batches and puree in a blender. If not, you can puree only half the soup and then mix it in with the rest to thicken the soup some.

Ladle the soup into bowls and garnish with a dollop of unsweetened vegan yogurt. Serves 8.

MEDITERRANEAN WHITE BEAN AND KALE SOUP

⅓ lb. dried white beans, soaked overnight

8 cups purified water or vegetable stock

2 bay leaves

2 tsp. sea salt, divided, or more to taste

2 Tbsp. extra-virgin olive oil

1½ cups yellow onion, chopped

4 garlic cloves, minced

1 cup fennel, chopped

1 cup celery, chopped

½ cup carrot, chopped

½ cup fresh parsley, chopped

¾ tsp. freshly ground black pepper

2 Tbsp. fresh oregano, chopped or 2 tsp. dried
    oregano

6 cups kale (about 2 bunches), chopped

¼ cup fresh basil, chopped

1 tsp. dried tarragon

4 cups vegetable stock (homemade if possible)

⅓ cup chickpea miso

3 Tbsp. nutritional yeast (optional)

Soak the beans overnight or quick soak them by bringing them to a boil for 1 minute, turning off the heat, covering them, and letting them soak in the warm water for 1–2 hours. Drain the beans and place them in a stock pot with the water or stock. Cover the beans and bring them to a boil. Remove the cover, lower the heat, and add bay leaves. Simmer for 40 minutes. Add 1 teaspoon of salt and continue to simmer until the beans are tender (about 10 minutes). Remove the beans from heat and allow to cool. Then take a large stock pot, add the oil, and heat over medium-low heat. Add the onions and garlic, and sauté until for 7–10 minutes or until the onions are clear. Add the fennel, celery, carrot, parsley, 2 pinches of salt, pepper, and oregano, and then cook until the vegetables are tender (about 7–10 minutes). Then add the kale, basil, and tarragon, and continue to cook for 7–10 minutes more, stirring occasionally.

When the beans are cool, drain them, reserving the liquid. Divide the beans and blend half with a small amount of the cooking liquid. Add the puree to the stockpot containing the vegetables, along with the whole beans. Next add 4 cups of the bean-cooking liquid and 4 cups of stock to the soup. Bring the soup to a boil, and then lower the heat to low and simmer for 20 minutes. Add a small amount of hot water to the miso and stir until it is thinned, and then add it to the soup along with the nutritional yeast. Stir and simmer for 5 minutes. Serves 6.

SOUTH OF THE BORDER BLACK BEAN SOUP

2 Tbsp. virgin coconut oil

1 large onion, chopped

3 garlic cloves, minced

6 cups water

2 cups black beans (soaked overnight, drained) or
   three 15-oz. cans black beans (drained)

1 cup fresh corn (cut off the cob) or frozen

½ cup red bell pepper, chopped

1 4½-oz. can diced green chilies or 2 Tbsp. diced
   mild green chile

¼ cup chopped cilantro

2 Tbsp. tomato paste

1 tsp. ground cumin

1 Tbsp. fresh oregano, chopped or 1 tsp. dried
   oregano

½ tsp. chili powder

Pinch fresh ground pepper

1 tsp. sea salt

Chopped cilantro for garnish (optional)

Minced onion for garnish (optional)

Place the coconut oil in a large stockpot and heat until the oil is melted. Then add the onion and garlic and sauté until they are tender. Then add the water and beans and continue heating until it boils. Then reduce the heat, cover, and let it simmer until the beans are tender (about 1½ hours). If you choose to use canned beans instead, simmer for 30 minutes.

After the soup has simmered, add the corn, red bell pepper, chilies, cilantro, tomato paste, cumin, oregano, chili powder, and black pepper and stir. Let it remain uncovered and simmering until the soup is thicker (about 30 minutes). For a thicker soup, let it simmer for a longer amount of time. If desired, you can separate the soup into batches and blend one batch and then stir it back in with the remainder of the soup to thicken the soup quickly. This will also make the soup creamier. (If you want to blend half the soup to thicken it, you may want to add the corn after it has been blended.) Once the soup is thickened, add salt and stir.

Serve in bowls and garnish if you choose. Serves 4–6.

TRI-BEAN COCONUT LIME TORTILLA SOUP

Created by Chef Jeff for this book, this is a delicious bean soup with a Mexican flare.

2 Tbsp. olive oil
1 large red onion, small diced
6 garlic cloves, minced
2 jalapeño peppers, small diced
1 15-oz. can black beans, drained and rinsed
1 15-oz. can pinto beans, drained and rinsed
1 15-oz. can kidney beans, drained and rinsed
1 14.5-oz. can crushed tomatoes
1 14.5-oz. can diced tomatoes (or 4 roma tomatoes, small diced)
1 14-oz. can unsweetened coconut milk

6 cups vegetable broth

1 Tbsp. ground ginger

1 Tbsp. ground cumin

1 Tbsp. ground turmeric

1 lb. corn kernels, fresh or frozen

¼ cup fresh cilantro, chopped

2 Tbsp. fresh lime juice (1 lime, juiced)

1 tsp. sea salt

½ Tbsp. freshly ground black pepper

4 tortillas, cut into strips (use gluten-free tortillas if
desired)

Avocado, chopped (optional, for garnish)

Put olive oil in a large pot over medium heat and add onion, garlic, and jalapeño pepper and cook until translucent, about 5 minutes. Add the beans, tomatoes, coconut milk, vegetable broth, ginger, cumin, and turmeric, and bring to a boil. Reduce heat and simmer for approximately 45 minutes. Then add the corn, cilantro, lime juice, salt, and pepper. Cook for another 5 minutes.

While the soup is cooking, prepare the tortilla garnish. Preheat oven to 375 degrees. Cut each tortilla in half, then cut each half into ¼-inch wide strips. Place the strips in a single layer on a baking sheet and sprinkle with salt, if desired. Bake for about 15 minutes, flipping every 5 minutes, until golden brown. Remove from oven and allow to cool uncovered until soup is ready. Garnish the soup with fresh cilantro and the baked tortilla strips. You can also garnish with chopped avocado, if desired. Serves 6–8.

YUMMY RED LENTIL SOUP

1 Tbsp. virgin coconut oil
1 cup onion, diced
1 cup green onions, diced
2–3 garlic cloves, minced or pressed
1 cup dry red lentils
7 cups purified water or vegetable stock (if using
    water, add 1 vegetable bouillon cube)
1 6-oz. can tomato paste
1 large tomato, chopped
1 Tbsp. fresh lemon juice (½ lemon, juiced)
4 cups chopped spinach
Sea salt and pepper to taste

Heat the oil in a small skillet on low heat. Add the onion, green onion, and garlic and sauté until onion is translucent. Place the lentils in a fine-mesh wire strainer and rinse well. In a soup kettle combine lentils and water (or vegetable stock). Bring the mixture to a boil, then skim off any foam that forms on the top of the lentils. Add the tomato paste, bouillon cube (if using water rather than vegetable stock), and the sautéed onion, green onion, and garlic. Reduce the heat and simmer for about 15 minutes. Add the chopped tomato, lemon juice, and chopped spinach along with the salt and pepper. Simmer for an additional 20–30 minutes or until lentils are tender. Serves 6.

ZESTY LENTIL SOUP WITH SPINACH

3 Tbsp. coconut oil

1½ tsp. ground cumin

1½ tsp. garam masala

¼ tsp. ground cloves

¾ tsp. sea salt

3 garlic cloves, minced

2 yellow onions, chopped

½ bunch celery, finely chopped

5 carrots, finely chopped

1 cup red lentils

1 cup baby spinach

2 bay leaves

8 cups vegetable stock

¼ cup fresh herb of choice (cilantro, basil, rosemary)

¼ tsp. sea salt

1 tsp. ground turmeric

1 Tbsp. red wine vinegar (optional)

In a large pot over medium-high heat melt the oil. Then add cumin, garam masala, cloves, and salt and stir for 15 seconds. Add the garlic, onion, celery, and carrots to the pot, and sauté the vegetables for 5–7 minutes. They should glisten when it is time to move on to the next step.

Add lentils, spinach, bay leaves, and stock. Stir as necessary to keep the lentils from sticking to the pot; bring the soup to a boil. Then turn heat to low, partially cover the pot, and simmer for 30 minutes, stirring occasionally.

Stir in fresh herbs, salt, and turmeric. Add red wine

vinegar if desired, or season with more salt to taste. Serves 4.

SOUPS WITH MUSCLE MEAT

ASIAN CHICKEN SOUP WITH COCONUT, LIME, AND GINGER

This is just like the coconut chicken soup you find at a Thai restaurant.

- 1 Tbsp. virgin coconut oil
- 1 medium shallot, sliced thin
- 1 garlic clove, minced
- 1½ Tbsp. lemongrass, minced
- 2 chilies, sliced thin
- 1 tsp. red curry paste
- 24 oz. chicken stock, preferably fresh
- 10 oz. full-fat coconut milk (if using canned milk, add 13.5 ounces and cut back a bit on the chicken stock)
- 1- to 2-inch-chunk galangal root (Thai ginger), sliced thin and bruised with the knife or 1- to 2-inch-chunk ginger, sliced thin
- 3 Tbsp. Thai fish sauce
- 2 roma tomatoes, seeded and diced
- 1 cup button mushrooms, cut into wedges
- 8 oz. skinless, boneless, free-range chicken breast, cut into ½-inch pieces
- 4 kaffir lime leaves, bruised
- 1 Tbsp. lime juice, or to taste (½ lime, juiced)

2 Tbsp. cilantro, chopped
¼ cup basil, chopped

In a heavy stockpot heat the oil and add the shallot, garlic, lemongrass, chilies, and red curry paste. Stir constantly for 30 seconds or until fragrant, but not burned.

Add chicken stock, coconut milk, galangal root (or ginger root), and fish sauce. Bring the soup to a boil, then reduce heat and simmer for 3 minutes.

Add tomatoes, mushrooms, chicken, and kaffir lime leaves. Turn the heat to low and simmer gently. Add lime juice, then remove the pot from heat. Remove galangal and kaffir lime leaves; garnish with cilantro and basil, as desired, and serve. Serves 4.

CHICKEN STOCK SUPREME

You can use cooked chicken or raw chicken to make stock. This chicken stock recipe is compliments of my friend Chef Jeff.

6–8 lb. chicken bones with some meat still attached
2 medium yellow onions, halved
3 carrots, chopped
3 ribs celery, coarsely chopped
3 bay leaves
1 Tbsp. fresh thyme or ½ Tbsp. dried thyme leaves
1 tsp. apple cider vinegar (optional)
1 tsp. ground peppercorns (optional)
¼ cup fresh parsley (optional)
Purified water

Put all ingredients into a stockpot and cover with purified water. The water should be 1–2 inches over the ingredients. Heat over medium-high heat and bring to a boil. Then reduce heat and let it simmer slowly. Remove any foam that appears on the top. Continue to let it simmer for 4–12 hours.

Remove the stock from heat and strain it. Let it cool and then pour it into containers for storage.

Stock can keep for 4–5 days in the refrigerator (longer if it is boiled for 10 minutes). This stock can also be frozen if you need it to keep for longer (up to several months). If you freeze it, make sure to leave room at the top of the container because the stock will expand.

If you refrigerate the stock, the fat will congeal at the top of the container. You can skim that off. The stock itself should have the consistency of Jell-O once chilled.

If you would prefer to use a Crock-Pot rather than the stove top to make stock, you can. Simply put all ingredients into the Crock-Pot and turn it on low and simmer for 6–12 hours.

Note: This basic recipe can be modified with turkey, beef, venison, or fish bones to make different types of stock.

CHICKEN VEGETABLE SOUP

This recipe makes a lot of soup, so it is best to make on the weekend and freeze batches of it for busy days.

  2 Tbsp. extra-virgin olive oil
  4 parsnips (about 1 lb.), cut into ½-inch pieces

4 ribs celery

1 turnip (about ¾ lb.), cut into ½-inch pieces

1 jalapeño pepper, seeded and chopped

1 Tbsp. garlic, chopped

2 tsp. sea salt

½ tsp. cayenne pepper

1 cup carrots, chopped

1 cup chard greens, chopped

1 cup green beans

1 10-oz. box frozen broccoli florets

1½ cup onion, chopped

16 cups chicken broth

¼ cup lemon juice (2 lemons, juiced)

1½ lb. (5 cups) cooked free-range chicken

¼ cup fresh dill, chopped, or 1 Tbsp. dried dill

Put oil in a large stockpot and heat over medium heat; then add the parsnips, celery, turnip, jalapeño pepper, garlic, salt, and cayenne pepper. Cook the vegetables until they are slightly tender but still crisp. Add the carrots, chard greens, green beans, broccoli, onion, chicken broth, lemon juice, chicken, and dill. Bring the soup to a boil and then reduce the heat and let it simmer for 5 minutes. Serves about 20.

JAMAICAN COCONUT CURRY CHICKEN SOUP

This recipe was created by Chef Jeff for this book.

2 Tbsp. olive oil

4 boneless, skinless chicken breasts, medium diced

1 large onion, small diced

6 garlic cloves, minced

1 jalapeño pepper, small diced

3 Tbsp. Jamaican curry powder

2 14-oz. cans unsweetened coconut milk

2 cups chicken broth

¼ cup fresh cilantro, chopped

1 tsp. sea salt

½ Tbsp. pepper

2 Tbsp. arrowroot in 4 Tbsp. cold water (mixed together until smooth)

1 cup freshly cooked white rice

Put olive oil in a large stockpot over medium heat and add chicken. Simmer for 5 minutes. Then add onion, garlic, and jalapeño pepper, and cook until translucent (about 5 minutes). Add the Jamaican curry powder, stir to combine, and cook for an additional 5 minutes. Then add the coconut milk and chicken broth and simmer for 1 hour (stir about every 10 minutes to avoid scorching on the bottom). Then add the cilantro, salt, pepper, and arrowroot. Let it simmer for a few minutes. You can mix all the rice into the soup. Serves 6.

QUICK TURKEY (OR VEGAN) CHILI

This recipe can either be made with ground turkey (or beef) or without meat for a vegan chili.

1 large yellow onion, chopped

1 green pepper, chopped

2 Tbsp. coconut oil

1 lb. ground beef or turkey (omit for vegan soup)

2 cans (4 cups) tomatoes

1–2 tsp. chili powder

1½ tsp. sea salt

3 large garlic cloves, finely chopped

1 bay leaf

Dash of paprika

Dash of cayenne pepper

¼ cup water, as needed

1 No. 2 can (2½ cups) red chili beans

In a large soup kettle or Dutch oven sauté onion and green pepper in coconut oil until tender, about 5 minutes on medium heat. In a separate pan, saute the meat until done. Add tomatoes and seasonings. Turn heat to low, add meat, and simmer for 2 hours. Add water, as necessary. Add beans and heat thoroughly. Serves 6.

TURKEY VEGETABLE SOUP

Make this soup for dinner and serve a bowl up for lunch the next day.

1½ lb. turkey thighs, skin removed

Water to cover (5–6 cups)

2 bay leaves

5 peppercorns

¼ cup parsley, chopped

2 ribs celery, chopped

1 cup jicama, cubed into ½-inch pieces

1 large yellow onion, quartered
1 large carrot, cut into ½-inch slices
1 cup zucchini, chopped
1 14-oz. can tomatoes, drained
1½ tsp. sea salt
1 tsp. garlic, minced
½ tsp. coarsely ground pepper
½ tsp. dried oregano
⅛ tsp. mace
1 cup wild rice, cooked

Place turkey thighs, water, bay leaves, peppercorns, parsley, and celery in a stockpot on high heat until it boils. Then cover the soup, put heat on low, and simmer. After 45 minutes, remove the bay leaves and discard them. Then remove turkey thighs, allow them to cool, and then trim the meat from the bones in large chunks. Throw away the bones and then place the meat back in the pot. Add the jicama, onion, carrot, zucchini, tomatoes, salt, garlic, pepper, oregano, and mace. Bring the soup back to a boil and then lower the heat and simmer until the vegetables are soft (about 30 minutes). Then add the cooked wild rice and simmer for another 10 minutes. Serves 6.

RESOURCES

CONNECT WITH CHERIE

Cherie's website

Go to www.juiceladycherie.com for information on juicing or weight loss. You can sign up for the Juicy Tips Newsletter to get recipes and healthy tips twice a week from America's most-trusted nutritionist. When you sign up, you will get a free recipe and 10 percent off your first order from Cherie's website.

You can also sign up for a five-day guided juice fast—The Juice Lady's Juice FASSST—on her website.

The Juice Lady's Health and Wellness Juice & Raw Foods Cleanse Retreats

You are invited to join us for a week that can change your life! Our retreats offer gourmet organic raw foods with a three-day juice fast midweek. We present interesting, informative classes in a beautiful, peaceful setting where you can experience healing and restoration of body and soul. For more information and dates for the retreats, visit http://www.juiceladycherie.com/Juice /juice-raw-food-retreat/ or call 866-843-8935.

The Juice Lady's 30-Day Detox Challenge

This is a four-week e-course designed to help your body get rid of toxins, contaminants, waste, and heavy metals that can accumulate in joints, organs, tissues, cells, the lymphatic system, and the bloodstream. It can energize your entire body. You'll get an e-lesson each week, private Facebook coaching with Cherie, and a teleconference call each week when you can ask questions. For more information, go to http://www.juiceladycherie.com /Juice/30-day-detox/ or call 866-843-8935.

The Juice Lady's 28-Day Juicing for Weight Loss

This four-week course has eight downloadable lessons to help you lose the weight you want. For more information go to www.juiceladycherie.com/Juice/juicing-for -weight-loss/ or call 866-843-8935.

Nutrition counseling

To schedule a nutrition consultation with the Juice Lady's team, visit http://www.juiceladycherie.com/Juice /nutritional-counseling/ or call 866-843-8935.

Scheduling Cherie Calbom to speak

To schedule Cherie Calbom to speak for your organization, call 866-843-8935.

BOOKS BY CHERIE AND JOHN CALBOM

These books can be ordered at Cherie's website or by calling 866-843-8935.

- Cherie Calbom, *The Juice Lady's Guide to Fasting* (Siloam)

- Cherie Calbom, *The Juice Lady's Remedies for Diabetes* (Siloam)

- Cherie Calbom, *Sugar Knockout* (Siloam)

- Cherie Calbom, Abby Fammartino, *The Juice Lady's Anti-Inflammation Diet* (Siloam)

- Cherie Calbom, *The Juice Lady's Big Book of Juices and Green Smoothies* (Siloam)

- Cherie Calbom, *The Juice Lady's Remedies for Asthma and Allergies* (Siloam)

- Cherie Calbom, *The Juice Lady's Remedies for Stress and Adrenal Fatigue* (Siloam)

- Cherie Calbom, *The Juice Lady's Weekend Weight-Loss Diet* (Siloam)

- Cherie Calbom, *The Juice Lady's Living Foods Revolution* (Siloam)

- Cherie Calbom, *The Juice Lady's Turbo Diet* (Siloam)

- Cherie Calbom, *The Juice Lady's Guide to Juicing for Health* (Avery)

- Cherie Calbom and John Calbom, *Juicing, Fasting, and Detoxing for Life* (Wellness Central)

- Cherie Calbom, *The Wrinkle Cleanse* (Avery)

- Cherie Calbom and John Calbom, *The Coconut Diet* (Wellness Central)

- Cherie Calbom, John Calbom, and Michael Mahaffey, *The Complete Cancer Cleanse* (Thomas Nelson)

- Cherie Calbom, *The Ultimate Smoothie Book* (Wellness Central)

CHERIE'S RECOMMENDATIONS

Juicers

To find out about the best juicers recommended by Cherie, call 866-843-8935 or visit www.juiceladycherie.com.

Dehydrators

To find out the best dehydrators recommended by Cherie, call 866-843-8935 or visit www.juiceladycherie.com.

Veggie powders and supplements

To purchase or get information on Sweet Wheat wheatgrass juice powder, go to www.juiceladycherie .com/Juice/products/#!/Supplements/c/4641363/offset=9 &sort=normal.

Garden's Best Genesis Superfood formula, available in powder and capsules, are ideal for when you travel or when you can't get juice made. You can also add it to your juices for extra nutrition. Go to www.juicelady cherie.com for more information or to purchase.

Internal cleansing kits

The complete and comprehensive Internal Cleanse Kit contains eighteen items for a twenty-one-day cleanse program, and with the free colon cleanse kit, you'll have a complete four-week cleanse program. You will get the colon-cleanse kit, along with Liver-Gallbladder Rejuvenator, Friendly Bacteria Replenisher, Lung Rejuvenator, Kidney and Bladder Rejuvenator, Blood and Skin Rejuvenator, and Lymph Rejuvenator. See the website for more information. You may order the cleansing products and get the 10 percent discount by calling 866-843-8935.

You can also find more information on other cleanse kits on the website. Along with the internal cleansing kit, there is a Colon Cleanse Kit, which contains Toxin Absorber (fiber and bentonite clay) and the herbal supplement Digestive Stimulator. There is also a Para Cleansing Kit, which contains herbs to help you get rid of parasites.

Lymphasizer (swing machine)

For cleansing and moving lymph, the lymphasizer is very helpful. The regular use of this relaxing massage movement stimulates the body, helps achieve stress reduction, and cleanses the lymphatic system. The swing machine is also referred to as a lymphasizer. Find it at www.juiceladycherie.com/Juice /products-2/#!/Swing-Machine-Lymphasizer/p/19801415 /category=4641818.

Berry Breeze

Keep your produce fresher longer and your fridge smelling fresh too. Berry Breeze can save you up to $2,200 a year from lost produce. Go to https://www.juicelady cherie.com/Juice//?s=berry+breeze for more information.

EmWave2

This is a cardiobiofeedback device. With it you can destress and learn heart-focused breathing. Find more information at www.juiceladycherie.com/Juice /products/#!/emWave®2/p/65101751/category=0.

Amino acid program

For brain neurotransmitter testing, go to neurogistics .com. Use my practitioner code SLEEP (all caps). You can order your brain neurotransmitter test there, and it will give you a recommendation of the amino acid supplements you need to balance your brain neurotransmitters.

NOTES

INTRODUCTION

1. Jeanette Settembre, "'The Soup Cleanse,' a New Cookbook, Helps You Lose Weight Fast," NYDailyNews.com, accessed March 16, 2017, http://www.nydailynews.com/life-style/eats/soup -cleansing-better-juicing-article-1.2481175.

CHAPTER 1
MY OWN JOURNEY TO HEALTH

1. "Quotations About Healthy Eating," Topend Sports, accessed March 16, 2017, http://www.top endsports.com/health/nutrition/quotes-food.htm.

CHAPTER 2
SOUP: THE ULTIMATE
COMFORT FOOD

1. Urvija Banerji, "The First Restaurants Only Served Soup," Atlas Obscura, May 10, 2016, accessed March 17, 2017, http://www.atlasobscura.com /articles/the-first-restaurants-only-served-soup.

2. Allison Siebecker, "Traditional Bone Broth in Modern Health and Disease," Townsend Letter for Doctors and Patients, February/March 2005, accessed March 16, 2017, http://www.townsend letter.com/FebMarch2005/broth0205.htm.

3. Louis P. DeGouy, *The Soup Book* (New York: Dover Publications, 1974).

4. Chris Reidy, "Campbell's Chicken Noodle Soup Is Celebrating its 80th Birthday," Boston Globe Media Partners LLC, January 16, 2014, accessed May 22, 2017, http://archive.boston.com/business /news/2014/01/16/campbell-chicken-noodle-soup -celebrating-its-birthday/An7sdBupEWwR6uv Ghsb9iO/story.html.

5. "French Onion Soup," ifood.tv, accessed March 17, 2017, http://ifood.tv/french/french-onion-soup /about.

6. John Edward Lind, "Dietetic Fads and Fancies," *International Record of Medicine and General Practice Clinics* 105 (1917): 889.

7. Charlotte Hilton Andersen, "8 Reasons to Try Bone Broth," Meredith Corporation, accessed May 22, 2017, http://www.shape.com/healthy-eating /cooking-ideas/8-reasons-try-bone-broth; Sarah Whitman, "What Are the Health Benefits of Eating Bone Marrow?" Leaf Group Ltd., updated April 17, 2015, accessed March 20, 2017, http:// www.livestrong.com/article/445905-what-are-the

-health-benefits-of-eating-bone-marrow/; Jacqueline Gabardy, "20 Amazing Benefits of Bone Broth," Sweet Beet and Green Bean, November 11, 2013, accessed May 21, 2017, http://sweetbeetandgreen bean.net/2013/11/11/20-amazing-benefits-of-bone -broth/.

8.   Laurie Colwin, *Home Cooking: A Writer in the Kitchen* (New York: Open Road Media, 2014).

9.   Louis P. De Gouy, *The Soup Book: Over 800 Recipes* (New York: Dover Publications, 1974).

CHAPTER 3
LIVING FOODS: THE
ESSENTIAL FOUNDATION

1.   "Julia Child Quotes," Goodreads Inc., accessed May 21, 2017, http://www.goodreads.com/quotes /814094-people-who-love-to-eat-are-always-the -best-people.

2.   Joseph Mercola, "McDonald's and Biophoton Deficiency," Mercola.com, August 21, 2002, accessed May 22, 2017, http://articles.mercola.com /sites/articles/archive/2002/08/21/biophoton.aspx.

3.   Ibid.

4.   Meg Campbell, "5 Things You Need to Know About the Health Benefits of Arugula," Leaf Group Ltd., updated April 19, 2016, accessed May 21, 2017, http://www.livestrong.com/article/5381 -need-health-benefits-arugula/; "The Top 10

Arugula Health Benefits," Superfood Profiles, accessed April 28, 2017, http://superfoodprofiles .com/arugula-health-benefits.

5. "17 Impressive Benefits of Asparagus," Organic Information Services Pvt Ltd., accessed April 28, 2017, https://www.organicfacts.net/health-benefits /vegetable/health-benefits-of-asparagus.html; "Asparagus," The George Mateljan Foundation, accessed April 28, 2017, http://www.whfoods.com /genpage.php?tname=foodspice&dbid=12.

6. "12 Benefits of Basil + Recipe Ideas," Draxe.com, accessed April 28, 2017, https://draxe.com/benefits -of-basil/; "What's So Healthy About Basil?," Pre- cision Nutrition, accessed May 22, 2017, http:// www.precisionnutrition.com/healthy-basil; "Basil," The George Mateljan Foundation, accessed May 22, 2017, http://www.whfoods.com/genpage.php ?tname=foodspice&dbid=85.

7. "Beets," The George Mateljan Foundation, accessed May 22, 2017, http://www.whfoods.com/genpage .php?tname=foodspice&dbid=49.

8. Catharine Paddock, "Does Beetroot Juice Lower Blood Pressure?" Medical News Today, July 20, 2016, accessed May 22, 2017, http://www.medical newstoday.com/articles/288229.php.

9. "What Are Beet Greens Good For?" Food Facts, accessed May 23, 2017, http://foodfacts.mercola .com/beet-greens.html; Reed Mangels, "Iron in

the Vegan Diet," The Vegetarian Resource Group, accessed April 27, 2017, http://www.vrg.org /nutrition/iron.php.

10. "Broccoli," The George Mateljan Foundation, accessed May 23, 2017, http://www.whfoods.com /genpage.php?tname=foodspice&dbid=9.

11. "Brussels Sprouts," The George Mateljan Foundation, accessed May 23, 2017, http://www .whfoods.com/genpage.php?tname=foodspice &dbid=10.

12. Liivi Hess, "Cabbage Vs. Chemo for Cancer?," The Alternative Daily, accessed May 23, 2017, http:// www.thealternativedaily.com/cabbage-versus -chemo-for-cancer-treatment/; "Cabbage," Whfoods .org, accessed May 23, 2017, http://whfoods.org /genpage.php?tname=foodspice&dbid=19.

13. Sandra Amalie Lacoppidan, Cecilie Kyro, Steffen Loft, et al. "Adherence to a Healthy Nordic Food Index Is Associated With a Lower Risk of Type-2 Diabetes—The Danish Diet, Cancer and Health Cohort Study," *Nutrients* 7, no. 10 (October 2015): 8633–8644.

14. "Carrots," Whfoods.org, accessed May 23, 2017, http://www.whfoods.org/genpage.php?tname =foodspice&dbid=21; "10 Impressive Benefits of Carrots," Organic Information Services Pvt Ltd., accessed May 23, 2017, https://www.organicfacts .net/health-benefits/vegetable/carrots.html.

15. Talwinder S. Kahlon, Mei-Chen M. Chiu, and Mary H. Chapman, "Steam Cooking Significantly Improves in vitro Bile Acid Binding of Beets, Eggplant, Asparagus, Carrots, Green Beans, And Cauliflower," *Nutrition Research* 27, no. 12 (December 2007): 750–755; "Cauliflower," The George Mateljan Foundation, accessed May 23, 2017, http://www.whfoods.com/genpage.php?tname =foodspice&dbid=13.

16. "Celery," Whfoods.org, accessed May 23, 2017, http://whfoods.org/genpage.php?tname=foodspice &dbid=14.

17. Megan Heimer, "Ditch the Table Salt, Not the Sodium," Natural News Network, March 7, 2011, accessed May 23, 2017, http://www.naturalnews .com/031608_table_salt_sodium.html#.

18. "Swiss Chard," Whfoods.org, accessed May 23, 2017, http://whfoods.org/genpage.php?tname =foodspice&dbid=16.

19. "Cilantro & Coriander Seeds," Whfoods.org, accessed May 23, 2017, http://whfoods.org /genpage.php?tname=foodspice&dbid=70.

20. Megan Ware, "Cilantro: Health Benefits, Facts, Research," MedicalNewsToday.com, September 1, 2016, accessed May 23, 2017, http://www.medical newstoday.com/articles/277627.php.

21. "12 Cilantro Benefits, Nutrition & Recipes," Dr. Axe, accessed May 23, 2017, https://draxe.com /cilantro-benefits/.

22. "Corn," Whfoods.org, accessed May 2, 2017, http:// whfoods.org/genpage.php?tname=foodspice &dbid=90.

23. "5 Wonderful Benefits of Cucumber," Organic Information Services Pvt Ltd., accessed May 23, 2017, https://www.organicfacts.net/health-benefits /vegetable/cucumber.html; "Cucumbers," The George Mateljan Foundation, accessed May 23, 2017, http://www.whfoods.com/genpage.php?tname =foodspice&dbid=42.

24. Christian Nordqvist, "Garlic: Health Benefits, Therapeutic Benefits," Medical News Today, September 15, 2015, accessed May 23, 2017, http:// www.medicalnewstoday.com/articles/265853.php.

25. "22 Health Benefits of Ginger Root You Simply Won't Believe," The Hearty Soul, accessed May 31, 2017, http://theheartysoul.com/ginger-benefits/; "Top 10 Benefits of Ginger," Organic Information Services Pvt Ltd., accessed May 31, 2017, https:// www.organicfacts.net/health-benefits/herbs-and -spices/ginger.html; "Natural Ways to Lower Your Cholesterol," Diabetes Self-Management, updated July 29, 2016, accessed May 31, 2017, https://www .diabetesselfmanagement.com/managing-diabetes

/complications-prevention/natural-ways-to-lower
-your-cholesterol/.

26. "Green Beans," The George Mateljan Foundation,
    accessed May 31, 2017, http://www.whfoods.com
    /genpage.php?tname=foodspice&dbid=134; "7
    Impressive Benefits of Green Beans," Organicfacts
    .net, accessed April 28, 2017, https://www.organic
    facts.net/health-benefits/vegetable/green-beans
    .html.

27. "Kale," The George Mateljan Foundation, accessed
    May 31, 2017, http://whfoods.org/genpage.php
    ?tname=foodspice&dbid=38.

28. "Healthy Food Trends—Beans and Legumes,"
    Medlineplus.gov, reviewed April 24, 2016,
    accessed May 31, 2017, https://medlineplus.gov
    /ency/patientinstructions/000726.htm.

29. "Lentils," The George Mateljan Foundation,
    accessed May 31, 2017, http://www.whfoods.com
    /genpage.php?tname=foodspice&dbid=52.

30. "11 Amazing Benefits of Stinging Nettles," Organic
    Information Services Pvt Ltd., accessed May 31,
    2017, https://www.organicfacts.net/health
    -benefits/herbs-and-spices/stinging-nettle.html;
    Kassie Vance, "Stinging Nettle," Herballegacy.com,
    accessed May 31, 2017, http://www.herballegacy
    .com/Vance_History.html; Nicki Wolf, "Nutrition
    of Stinging Nettles," Lead Group Ltd., updated
    September 15, 2015, accessed May 31, 2017, http://

www.livestrong.com/article/350785-stinging
-nettles-nutrition/; Dalene Barton-Schuster, "How
to Use Fertility Herbs to Enhance Your Fertility Naturally," The Natural Fertility Company,
accessed May 31, 2017, http://natural-fertility-info
.com/fertility-herbs.

31. "Onions," The George Mateljan Foundation,
accessed May 31, 2017, http://whfoods.org
/genpage.php?tname=foodspice&dbid=45.

32. "Oregano," The George Mateljan Foundation,
accessed May 31, 2017, http://www.whfoods.com
/genpage.php?tname=foodspice&dbid=73;
"Fighting Free Radicals & Free Radical Damage,"
Dr.Axe.com, accessed May 31, 2017, https://draxe
.com/fighting-free-radical-damage/; Samina Kausar,
"Herbal Remedies for Throat Phlegm or Mucus,"
HealthnFairness.com, accessed May 31, 2017,
http://www.healthnfairness.com/2014/03/herbal
-remedies-for-throat-phlegm-or.html.

33. Andrew Chevallier, *Encyclopedia of Herbal Medicine*,
3rd ed. (New York: DK Publishing, 2016), 246; "7
Wonderful Parsley Health Benefits," Organicfacts
.net, accessed April 28, 2017, https://www.organic
facts.net/health-benefits/herbs-and-spices/health
-benefits-of-parsley.html.

34. "Green Peas," The George Mateljan Foundation,
accessed May 31, 2017, http://www.whfoods.com
/genpage.php?tname=foodspice&dbid=55; "10

Health Benefits of Peas," Real Food for Life, accessed May 31, 2017, http://www.realfoodforlife .com/10-health-benefits-of-peas/.

35. "11 Impressive Benefits of Rosemary," Organic Information Services Pvt Ltd., accessed May 31, 2017, https://www.organicfacts.net/health-benefits /herbs-and-spices/rosemary.html; "11 Surprising Health Benefits of Rosemary and Its Memorable Flavor," Your Health Tube, September 22, 2016, accessed May 31, 2017, http://yourhealthtube.com /11-health-benefits-rosemary-memorable-flavor/.

36. "Spinach," The George Mateljan Foundation, accessed May 31, 2017, http://www.whfoods.com /genpage.php?tname=foodspice&dbid=43; Tracey Roizman, "Does Chlorophyll Cleanse the Blood?," Livestrong.com, September 12, 2011, accessed May 31, 2017, http://www.livestrong.com/article/542432 -does-chlorophyll-cleanse-the-blood/.

37. "7 Amazing Thyme Benefits," Organic Information Services Pvt Ltd., accessed May 31, 2017, https:// www.organicfacts.net/health-benefits/herbs-and -spices/thyme.html; Adam Fonseca, "Uses of Thymol," Livestrong.com, July 27, 2015, accessed May 31, 2017, http://www.livestrong.com/article /163688-uses-of-thymol/; Juliana DeCarvalho Anderson, "Ebers Papyrus," Toxipedia, July 25, 2012, accessed May 16, 2017, http://www.toxipedia .org/display/toxipedia/Ebers+Papyrus; "Thyme," The George Mateljan Foundation, accessed May 31,

2017, http://whfoods.org/genpage.php?tname
=foodspice&dbid=77.

38. S. A. Lazarus, K. Bowen, and M. L. Garg,
"Tomato Juice and Platelet Aggregation in Type
2 Diabetes," *Journal of the American Medical Association* 292, no. 7 (August 18, 2004): 805–806;
"Tomatoes," The George Mateljan Foundation,
accessed May 31, 2017, http://whfoods.org
/genpage.php?tname=foodspice&dbid=44.

39. Megan Ware, "Watercress: Health Benefits and
Nutritional Breakdown," Healthline Media UK
Ltd., updated October 20, 2016, accessed May 31,
2017, http://www.medicalnewstoday.com/articles
/285412.php.

40. Lizette Borelli, "Benefits of Watercress: Lower
Blood Pressure and 5 Other Conditions It Can
Alleviate," Newsweek Media Group, October 3,
2016, accessed May 31, 2017, http://www.medical
daily.com/benefits-watercress-lower-blood-pressure
-and-6-other-conditions-it-can-399859.

41. Ibid.

42. Ibid.

43. Ibid.

44. Ibid.

45. "5 Amazing Zucchini Benefits," Organic Information Services Pvt Ltd., accessed May 31, 2017,

https://www.organicfacts.net/health-benefits
/vegetable/health-benefits-of-zucchini.html; "Zucchini Nutrition—Low in Calories & Loaded
With Anti-Inflammatory Properties," Dr.Axe.com,
accessed May 31, 2017, https://draxe.com/zucchini
-nutrition/.

46. S. Sarkar and D. Buha, "Effect of Ripe Fruit
    Pulp Extract of Cucurbita Pepo Linn. in Aspirin
    Induced Gastric and Duodenal Ulcer in Rats,"
    Indian Journal of Experimental Biology 46, no. 9
    (October 2008): 639–645.

CHAPTER 4
DETOXING WITH SOUP

1. Kate DiCamillo, *The Tale of Despereaux* (Somer-
   ville, MA: Candlewick Press, 2009).

2. Cherie Calbom, *Juicing, Fasting, and Detoxing
   for Life* (New York: Grand Central Life & Style,
   2014), 132.

3. Cherie Calbom, *The Juice Lady's Guide to Juicing for
   Health* (New York: Penguin, 2008), 323.

4. Ibid., 310–311.

5. Ibid., 314.

6. "Turmeric," University of Maryland Medical
   Center, reviewed June 26, 2014, accessed April 4,
   2017, http://umm.edu/health/medical/altmed/herb
   /turmeric.

CHAPTER 5
A "SOUPER"
WEIGHT-LOSS SOLUTION

1. "Auguste Escoffier," AZ Quotes, accessed June 1, 2017, http://www.azquotes.com/quote/797292.

2. "How I Lost 11 Pounds in 7 Days With the Cabbage Soup Diet (and How You Can, Too)!," accessed June 1, 2017, http://www.cabbage-soup -diet.com/diet/.

3. Yong Zhu and James H. Hollis, "Soup Consumption Is Associated With a Reduced Risk of Overweight and Obesity but Not Metabolic Syndrome in US Adults: NHANES 2003–2006," *PLOS ONE* 8, no. 9 (2013), http://dx.doi.org/10.1371 /journal.pone.0075630.

4. Julie E. Flood and Barbara J. Rolls, "Soup Preloads in a Variety of Forms Reduce Meal Energy Intake," *Appetite* 49, no. 3 (November 2007): 626– 634, https://www.ncbi.nlm.nih.gov/pmc/articles /PMC2128765/.

5. Jack Challoner, "How Soup Can Help You Lose Weight," BBC, updated May 26, 2009, accessed June 1, 2017, http://news.bbc.co.uk/2/hi/uk_news /magazine/8068733.stm.

6. Ibid.

7. Richard Mattes, "Soup and Satiety," *Physiology & Behavior* 83, no. 5 (January 17, 2005): 739–747, https://doi.org/10.1016/j.physbeh.2004.09.021.

8. Barbara J. Rolls et al., "Provision of Foods Differing in Energy Density Affects Long-Term Weight Loss," *Obesity* 13, no. 6 (June 2005): 1052–1060. doi: 10.1038/oby.2005.123.

9. Maureen K. Spill et al., "Serving Large Portions of Vegetable Soup at the Start of a Meal Affected Children's Energy and Vegetable Intake," *Appetite* 57, no. 1 (August 2011): 213–219. doi: 10.1016/j.appet.2011.04.024.

10. Flood and Rolls, "Soup Preloads in a Variety of Forms Reduce Meal Energy Intake."

11. Mattes, "Soup and Satiety."

12. Ibid.

13. Barbara J. Rolls, Elizabeth A. Bell, and Michelle L. Thorwart, "Water Incorporated Into a Food but Not Served With a Food Decreases Energy Intake in Lean Women," *American Journal of Clinical Nutrition*, 70, no. 4 (October 1999): 448–455, http://ajcn.nutrition.org/content/70/4/448.full.pdf+html.

14. Challoner, "How Soup Can Help You Lose Weight."

15. Ana M Andrade, Geoffrey W. Greene, and Kathleen J. Meleanson, "Eating Slowly Led to Decreases in Energy Intake Within Meals in Healthy Women," *Journal of the American Dietetic Association* 108, no. 7 (July 2008): 1186–1191, http://www.sciencedirect.com/science/article/pii /S000282230800518X.

16. Flood and Rolls, "Soup Preloads in a Variety of Forms Reduce Meal Energy Intake."

17. *Dietary Guidelines for Americans 2010*, US Department of Agriculture and US Department of Health and Human Services, December 2010, accessed June 1, 2017, https://health.gov /dietaryguidelines/2010/.

18. A. Medina-Ramón et al., "Gazpacho Consumption Is Associated With Lower Blood Pressure and Reduced Hypertension in a High Cardiovascular Risk Cohort. Cross-Sectional Study of the PREDIMED Trial," *Nutrition, Metabolism and Cardiovascular Diseases* 23, no. 10 (October 2013): 944–952, https://www.ncbi.nlm.nih.gov/pubmed /23149074.

19. Barbara O. Rennard et al., "Chicken Soup Inhibits Neutrophil Chemotaxis *In Vitro*," *Chest* 118, no. 4 (2000), http://journal.publications.chestnet.org /article.aspx?articleid=1079188; K. Saketkhoo, A. Januszkiewicz, and M. A. Sackner, "Effects of Drinking Hot Water, Cold Water, and Chicken

Soup on Nasal Mucus Velocity and Nasal Airflow Resistance," *Chest* 74, no. 4 (October 1978): 408–410, https://www.ncbi.nlm.nih.gov/pubmed/359266.

20. Yong Zhu and James Hollis, "Soup Consumption Is Associated With a Lower Dietary Energy Density and a Better Diet Quality in US Adults," *British Journal of Nutrition* 111, no. 8 (April 2014): 1474–1480, https://www.cambridge.org/core/journals/british-journal-of-nutrition/article/soup-consumption-is-associated-with-a-lower-dietary-energy-density-and-a-better-diet-quality-in-us-adults/878E630DD29562D3CE48CEAC0C34FC03.

21. "Campbell's Chunky New England Clam Chowder Soup: Nutrition Facts," Hy-Vee Inc., accessed June 1, 2017, https://www.hy-vee.com/grocery/PD523600/Campbells-Chunky-New-England-Clam-Chowder-Soup.

22. "Consuming Canned Soup Linked to Greatly Elevated Levels of the Chemical BPA," The President and Fellows of Harvard College, November 22, 2011, accessed June 1, 2017, https://www.hsph.harvard.edu/news/press-releases/canned-soup-bpa/.

23. "The Watercress Soup Diet: Week One," Associated Newspapers Ltd., accessed June 1, 2017, http://www.dailymail.co.uk/health/article-112665/The-Watercress-Soup-diet-week-one.html.

24. Ibid.

25. "White Button Mushrooms in Place of Meat Can Help With Weight Loss," ScienceBlog.com, April 22, 2013, accessed June 1, 2017, https://scienceblog .com/62485/white-button-mushrooms-in-place-of -meat-can-help-with-eight-loss/.

26. A. B. Crujeiras et al., "A Hypocaloric Diet Enriched in Legumes Specifically Mitigates Lipid Peroxidation in Obese Subjects," *Free Radical Research* 41, no. 4 (April 2007): 498-506, https:// www.ncbi.nlm.nih.gov/pubmed/17454132.

27. M. A. Wien et al., "Almonds vs Complex Carbo-hydrates in a Weight Reduction Program," *International Journal of Obesity* 27 (2003): 1365–1371, http://www.nature.com/ijo/journal/v27/n11/abs /0802411a.html.

28. "Brain Chemical Boosts Body Heat, Aids in Cal-orie Burn, UT Southwestern Research Suggests," ScienceDaily, UT Southwestern Medical Center, July 7, 2010, accessed June 1, 2017, https://www .sciencedaily.com/releases/2010/07/100706123015 .htm.

29. "52 Thermogenic Foods That Naturally Burn Calo-ries as You Eat Them," HomeGymr, accessed June 1, 2017, http://homegymr.com/thermogenic-foods -list/.

30. Frank Yemi, "The Benefits of Garlic and Ginger in Losing Weight," Livestrong, updated June 17, 2015, accessed June 1, 2017, http://www.livestrong.com /article/538326-the-benefits-of-garlic-ginger-in -losing-weight/.

31. Jenny Hills, "How to Lose Weight and Belly Fat with Ginger (Research Based)," Healthy and Natural World, accessed June 1, 2017, http://www .healthyandnaturalworld.com/lose-weight-and -belly-fat-with-ginger/.

32. Musarrat Bano, "Natural Thermogenic Spices and Herbs for Losing Belly Fat," Natural Fitness Tips, March 1, 2017, accessed June 1, 2017, http://www .nftips.com/2013/12/natural-thermogenic-spices -and-herbs.html.

33. Ibid.

CHAPTER 6
THE HEALING POWER OF SOUP

1. John Steinbeck, *East of Eden* (New York: Penguin, 1952).

2. Rosie Schwartz, "Nutrition: The Health Benefits of Soup," ParentsCanada.com, November 15, 2013, accessed June 1, 2017, http://www.parentscanada .com/food/nutrition-the-health-benefits-of-soup.

3. Kasandra Brabaw, "5 Veggies That Are Healthier Cooked Than Raw," Rodale Inc., June 15, 2016, accessed March 30, 2017, http://www.prevention

.com/food/5-veggies-that-are-healthier-cooked
-than-raw.

4.   Diana Parsell, "Vegetable Soup Fights Cell
     Damage," Science News, November 9, 2004,
     accessed June 1, 2017, https://www.sciencenews
     .org/blog/food-thought/vegetable-soup-fights-cell
     -damage.

5.   Ibid.

6.   Ibid.

7.   Ibid.

8.   Ibid.

9.   Ibid.

10. "The Health Benefits of Mushroom Consumption,"
     Dr. Joseph Mercola, May 13, 2013, accessed June
     1, 2017, http://articles.mercola.com/sites/articles
     /archive/2013/05/13/mushroom-benefits.aspx.

11. Melissa Schorr, "Chicken Soup Really Is Good
     for a Cold," ABC News, accessed April 25, 2017,
     http://abcnews.go.com/Health/story?id=117888
     &page=1.

12. Saketkhoo, Januszkiewicz, and Sackner, "Effects
     of Drinking Hot Water, Cold Water, and Chicken
     Soup on Nasal Mucus Velocity and Nasal Airflow
     Resistance."

13. Jack Challem, "Natural Non-Drug Remedies for Inflammation," Khalsa Chiropractic, 2000, accessed June 1, 2017, http://www.drmhaatma.com /Q-inflamationsupplements.html.

14. Ann Bode and Zigang Dong, "The Amazing and Mighty Ginger," in *Herbal Medicine: Biomelecular and Clinical Aspects*, 2nd edition (Boca Raton, Florida: CRC Press, 2011); G. Ozgoli, M. Goli, and F. Moattar, "Comparison of Effects of Ginger, Mefenamic Acid, and Ibuprofen on Pain in Women With Primary Dysmenorrhea," *Journal of Alternative and Complementary Medicine* 15, no. 2 (2009):129–132.

15. Jane E. Brody, "A New Look at an Ancient Remedy: Celery," *New York Times*, June 9, 1992, accessed June 1, 2017, http://www.nytimes.com /1992/06/09/health/a-new-look-at-an-ancient -remedy-celery.html; "Celery Seed," University of Maryland Medical Center, reviewed June 22, 2015, accessed June 1, 2017, http://www.umm.edu/health /medical/altmed/herb/celery-seed.

16. Chris Kresser, "The Bountiful Benefits of Bone Broth: A Comprehensive Guide," Chriskresser.com, February 21, 2017, accessed June 1, 2017, https:// chriskresser.com/the-bountiful-benefits-of-bone -broth-a-comprehensive-guide/.

CHAPTER 7
HOW DO I BEGIN?

1. "Benjamin Franklin," AZ Quotes, accessed June 1, 2017, http://www.azquotes.com/quote/461875.

2. Chris Klint, "Once Again, Testing Finds Alaska Seafood Free of Fukushima Radiation," Alaska Dispatch Publishing, January 10, 2017, accessed June 1, 2017, https://www.adn.com/alaska-news /science/2017/01/10/once-again-testing-finds -alaska-seafood-free-of-fukushima-radiation/.

3. Sally Fallon and Mary G. Enig, "Newest Research on Why You Should Avoid Soy," Mercola.com, accessed May 16, 2017, http://www.mercola.com /article/soy/avoid_soy.htm; Peter Curcio, "Dissecting Anti-Nutrients: The Good and Bad of Phytic Acid," Breakingmuscle.com, accessed June 1, 2017, https://breakingmuscle.com/fuel /dissecting-anti-nutrients-the-good-and-bad-of -phytic-acid.

4. Chensheng Lu, Kathryn Toepel, Rene Irish, Richard Fenske, Dana Barr, and Roberto Bravo, "Organic Diets Significantly Lower Children's Dietary Exposure to Organophosphorus Pesticides," *Environmental Health Perspectives* 114, no. 2 (February 2006), https://www.ncbi.nlm.nih.gov/pmc /articles/PMC1367841/#__ffn_sectitle.

5. F. N. Chaudhry and M. F. Malik, "Factors Affecting Water Pollution: A Review," *Journal of Ecosystem and Ecography* 7, no. 1 (February 2017).

6. Allison Aubrey, "Is Organic More Nutritious? New Study Adds to the Evidence," NPR.org, February 18, 2016, accessed June 1, 2017, http://www.npr .org/sections/thesalt/2016/02/18/467136329/is -organic-more-nutritious-new-study-adds-to-the -evidence.

7. David Gutierrez, "Eating Organic Foods Reduces Pesticide Exposure by Nearly 90% After Just One Week," Natural News Network, May 6, 2014, accessed June 1, 2017, http://www.naturalnews .com/045006_organic_foods_pesticide_exposure _phthalates.html.

8. "Dirty Dozen," accessed June 1, 2017, https://www .ewg.org/foodnews/dirty_dozen_list.php.

9. "Clean Fifteen," accessed June 1, 2017, https://www .ewg.org/foodnews/clean_fifteen_list.php.

10. Lola Milholland, "Questions About Mexican Organics?," PCC Natural Markets, January 2011, accessed June 1, 2017, http://www.pccnatural markets.com/sc/1101/sc1101-mexican-organics .html.

11. Ibid.

12. Ibid.

13. G. Löfroth, "Toxic Effects of Irradiated Foods," *Nature* 211, no. 302 (July 1966).

14. "Food Irradiation: Hearing Before the Subcommittee on Health and the Environment of the Committee on Energy and Commerce, House of Representatives, One Hundredth Congress, First Session on H.R. 956," June 19, 1987, Volume 4 (Washington, DC: U.S. Government Printing Office, 1988); G. Löfroth, "Toxic Effects of Irradiated Foods," *Nature* 211, no. 302 (July 1966).

15. "Grocery Manufacturers Association Position on GMOs," The Grocery Manufacturers Association, accessed June 2, 2017, https://factsaboutgmos.org /disclosure-statement.

16. "10 Reasons to Avoid GMOs," Institute for Responsible Technology, August 25, 2011, accessed June 1, 2017, http://responsibletechnology.org/10 -reasons-to-avoid-gmos/.

17. Joseph Mercola, "Eating This Could Turn Your Gut Into a Living Pesticide Factory," TheHuffingtonPost.com Inc., January 29, 2013, accessed June 2, 2017, http://www.huffingtonpost.com/dr -mercola/bt-corn_b_2442072.html.

18. Joël Spiroux de Vendômois et al., "A Comparison of the Effects of Three GM Corn Varieties on Mammalian Health," *International Journal of Biological Sciences* 5, no. 7 (2009): 706–726, doi:10.7150/ijbs.5.706.

19. David Derbyshire, "Fears Grow as Study Shows Genetically Modified Crops 'Can Cause Liver and Kidney Damage,'" Associated Newspapers Ltd., January 21, 2010, accessed June 2, 2017, http://www.dailymail.co.uk/news/article-1244824/Fears-grow-study-shows-genetically-modified-crops-cause-liver-kidney-damage.html.

20. Spiroux de Vendômois et al., "A Comparison of the Effects of Three GM Corn Varieties on Mammalian Health."

21. "10 Reasons to Avoid GMOs," Institute for Responsible Technology.

22. Ibid.

23. Deborah B. Whitman, "Genetically Modified Foods: Harmful or Helpful?," CSA Discovery Guides, April 2000, accessed June 2, 2017, https://biomed.brown.edu/arise/resources/docs/GM%20foods%20review.pdf.

24. James E. McWilliams, "The Green Monster," TheSlateGroup, January 28, 2009, accessed June 2, 2017, http://www.slate.com/id/2209168/pagenum/all/; "9 Ingredients to Watch," Green America, April/May 2012, accessed June 2, 2017, https://www.greenamerica.org/pubs/greenamerican/articles/AprilMay2012/9-GM-ingredients-to-watch.cfm.

CHAPTER 8
SOUP RECIPES TO CLEANSE
YOUR BODY, ENCOURAGE
WEIGHT LOSS, RESTORE HEALTH,
AND INCREASE ENERGY

1. This recipe is adapted from Dr. Oz's Green Mung Bean Soup, found here: http://www.doctoroz.com /recipe/green-mung-bean-soup.

2. "Turmeric," University of Maryland Medical Center, reviewed June 26, 2014, accessed June 2, 2017, http://umm.edu/health/medical/altmed/herb /turmeric.

CONNECT WITH US!

CHARISMA HOUSE

(Spiritual Growth)

f Facebook.com/CharismaHouse

𝕏 @CharismaHouse

◉ Instagram.com/CharismaHouse

SILOAM

(Health)

𝓟 Pinterest.com/CharismaHouse

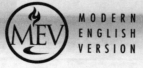

MODERN ENGLISH VERSION

(Bible)
www.mevbible.com

Ignite Your SPIRITUAL HEALTH with these FREE Newsletters

CHARISMA HEALTH
Get information and news on health-related topics and studies, and tips for healthy living.

POWER UP! FOR WOMEN
Receive encouraging teachings that will empower you for a Spirit-filled life.

CHARISMA MAGAZINE NEWSLETTER
Get top-trending articles, Christian teachings, entertainment reviews, videos and more.

CHARISMA NEWS WEEKLY
Get the latest breaking news from an evangelical perspective every Monday.

SIGN UP AT:
nl.charismamag.com

CHARISMA MEDIA